Medicare Now and in the Future
Second Edition

MARILYN MOON

Medicare Now and in the Future

Second Edition

THE URBAN INSTITUTE PRESS
Washington, D.C.

Library of Congress Cataloging in Publication Data

Medicare Now and in the Future, Second Edition/Marilyn Moon.

1. Medicare.   2.   Medicare—Forecasting.   3.   Medicare—Cost control.
4.   Forecasting.   5.   Medicare—trends.   I.   Title.

HD7102.U4M666   1993   92-38302
368.4′26′00973—dc20   CIP

ISBN 0-87766-653-9 (paper, alk. paper)

Printed in the United States of America.

Distributed in North America by
National Book Network
4720 Boston Way
Lanham, MD 20706

THE URBAN INSTITUTE is a nonprofit policy research and educational organization established in Washington, D.C., in 1968. Its staff investigates the social and economic problems confronting the nation and public and private means to alleviate them. The Institute disseminates significant findings of its research through the publications program of its Press. The goals of the Institute are to sharpen thinking about societal problems and efforts to solve them, improve government decisions and performance, and increase citizen awareness of important policy choices.

Through work that ranges from broad conceptual studies to administrative and technical assistance, Institute researchers contribute to the stock of knowledge available to guide decision making in the public interest.

Conclusions or opinions expressed in Institute publications are those of the authors and do not necessarily reflect the views of staff members, officers or trustees of the Institute, advisory groups, or any organizations that provide financial support to the Institute.

CONTENTS

Foreword   xiii

Preface   xv

1 Placing Medicare in Context   1
Why Examine Medicare Now?   2
Economic Status of Older Americans   5
  Prospects for the Future   9
  Burdens from Health Spending   10
The Economic Status of Disabled Persons   13
The Problem of Rising Healthcare Costs   13
  Prices   14
  Use of Services   16
Medicare as Part of Federal Budget   20
The Specific Financing Issues Facing Medicare   21
Rethinking Medicare Policy   22

2 Assuring Access   27
The Genesis   28
  Evolution of the Legislation   28
  Medicare and Its Goals   31
Expansion in 1972   33
Other Changes in Access   35
Who Gets What?   37
  Rising Burdens of Medicare Cost Sharing   38
  Geographic Variation   41
Conclusions   42

3 Containing Costs: Impacts on Providers   45
Sources of Growth in Medicare Spending   46
Changing Medicare's Relationship with Providers   51
Hospitals Take the First Hit   52

How PPS Works   55
The Immediate Response in Delivery of Care   59
Impacts on Hospitals   60
Impact on Medicare Administration   66
Changes to Improve Hospital Payment   68
Physician Payment Reform   69
Details of the Medicare Fee Schedule   73
The Impact of the Fee Schedule   76
Other Provider Changes   78
Home Health Services   78
Skilled Nursing Facility Care   81
Health Maintenance Organizations   82
Conclusions   84

4 Containing Costs: Impacts on Beneficiaries   89
Direct Changes in Beneficiary Cost Sharing   90
Sources of Higher Beneficiary Burdens   91
Offsetting Reductions in Beneficiary Burdens   93
Distribution of the Impact   97
PPS and Indirect Burdens on Beneficiaries   99
Effects of Shorter Hospital Stays   100
Shifting the Site of Service   103
Effects of Less Inpatient Care   103
Quality of Care   104
Medicare Physician Payment Reform and Quality   105
HMOs and Quality   106
Peer Review Organizations   107
Using Effectiveness Studies to Improve Quality   108
Program Satisfaction   109
Conclusions   111

5 The Medicare Catastrophic Coverage Act   115
Recognizing the Need for Catastrophic Protection   116
Setting the Stage for the Legislation   118
Evolution of the Legislation   118
Defining the Benefits   119
Financing   121
The Medicare Catastrophic Coverage Act: Passage and Repeal   122
Overall Beneficiary Impact   127
Winners and Losers   128
The Beginning of the End   131
Repeal   133

Lessons for Health Policy   134
    Politics of the Supplemental Premium   135
    Lessons for Medicare's Future   137
Conclusions   141

6 Marginal Changes and the Future   145
Restructuring Cost Sharing   145
Cost-Containment Strategies   148
    Hospitals   150
    Physicians   153
    Other Changes in Provider Payments   154
    HMOs and Other Managed-Care Approaches   155
    Effectiveness Studies   157
    Cuts Directed at Beneficiaries   159
Modest Benefit Expansions   164
    Administrative Simplifications   165
    Hospice Care and the Last Year of Life   166
    Preventive Services   168
Conclusions   169

7 Reducing the Cost of Medicare   173
Shifting Risks   174
    Balancing Choice and Risk   174
    Vouchers   176
    Capitated Care Options   179
Reducing Coverage   181
    Making Medicare the Insurer of Last Resort   181
    Substantially Increasing Medicare's Premium   183
    Taxing the Value of Medicare Benefits   185
Limiting Eligibility   187
    Increasing the Age of Eligibility   188
    Age Rationing   189
    Means Testing Medicare   192
Conclusions   193

8 Expanding Medicare   197
Improving Acute Care   197
    Moving an Expanded QMB Program to Medicare   198
    Adding Stop-Loss Protection   199
    Expanding Eligibility for Medicare   200
    Adding a Prescription Drug Benefit to Medicare   204

Adding Long-Term Care   205
    Comprehensive Long-Term Care Coverage   206
    An Income-Related Benefit   209
    Limited Expansion of Medicare Benefits for Long-Term Care   209
    Changing the Composition of Medicare Services   211
    An Optional Long-Term Care Benefit   212
Conclusions   215

9 How Should Medicare Change?   219
Factors Constraining Medicare Reforms   220
First Steps   223
    Continue Efforts at Cost Containment Involving Providers   223
    Modestly Expand Managed Care Options   224
    Revise Cost Sharing   226
    Expand the Part B Premium   228
    Expand the QMB Program   229
    Expand the Hospice Program   230
    Streamline Billing and Administration   231
Longer Term Steps   232
    Further Reform Medicare to Address Costs of Healthcare   232
    Increase Direct Costs to Beneficiaries   233
    Increase Public Financing for Medicare   234
    Improve Acute-Care Coverage   235
    Expand Long-Term Care Coverage   236
Conclusions   237

Appendix   241

References   257

About the Author   261

Index   263

Tables
1.1   Growth in Median Income for all Elderly and for Specific Cohort
      in the United States, 1985–90   6
1.2   Average Family Income of Older Americans by Quintile, 1992   8
1.3   Health Care Spending Out-of-Pocket and on Premiums as Share
      of Income   11
2.1   Components of Medicare Cost Sharing, 1993   38

2.2   Average Annual per Capita Cost of Medicare for Persons Aged
      65 + for Selected Counties, 1996   42
3.1   Average Annual Percentage Changes in Medicare, 1967–93   47
3.2   Most Common DRGs and Their Weights   57
3.3   Rate of Change in Hospital Admissions for Medicare Enrollees,
      1980–91   62
3.4   Distribution of PPS Operating Margins, by Hospital Group, PPS
      10   65
3.5   Change in Payment and Use per Beneficiary for Selected
      Services, 1992–95   77
3.6   Medicare Beneficiaries Enrolled in HMOs   83
4.1   Sources of Increased Enrollee Liability for Medicare Benefits,
      1991   91
4.2   Use of Medicare Services for 1,000 Medicare Enrollees, by Age:
      1993   97
4.3   Variations in Medicare Out-of-Pocket Liabilities, by Age, 1993   98
5.1   Proportion of Elderly in the United States with Out-of-Pocket
      Spending More Than 15 Percent of Income, by Income and
      Hospital Use, 1986   117
5.2   Medicare Catastrophic Coverage Act Benefits as Enacted in 1988   124
5.3   Medicare Benefit Payments, Copayment Liabilities, and
      Premiums Payable per Enrollee Before and After
      Implementation of Medicare Catastrophic Coverage Act of
      1988   128
5.4   Net Change in Enrollees' Out-of-Pocket Costs by Income and
      Poverty Status in Response to Medicare Catastrophic
      Coverage Act of 1988   130
6.1   Budget Neutral Options for Restructuring Cost Sharing of
      Medicare   147
6.2   Options for Restructuring Cost Sharing of Medicare for about $5
      Billion in Federal Savings in 1996   160
7.1   Estimated Revenue Increases as a Share of Current Part B
      Premium from Income-Related Options, 1996   186
7.2   Options for Achieving Medicare Savings   194

Figures
1.1   Medicare as Share of Federal Budget, 1965–95   3
1.2   Annual Federal Outlays for Medicare, 1967–2000   4
1.3   Poverty Rates in the United States for Persons Aged 65 and
      Older, 1966–94   7
1.4   Health Insurance Supplementing Medicare: 1991   11
1.5   Healthcare Price Inflation in the United States, 1970–95   15

1.6   Average Annual Growth Rates in Physician Net Income by
       Specialty in the United States, 1979–88   16
1.7   Per Capita Growth Rates of Services Covered by Both Medicare
       and Private Insurance   19
1.8   HI Trust Fund Assets at End of the Year, in Billions   23
2.1   Annual Percentage Change in Number of Medicare Enrollees:
       CY 1967–93   35
2.2   Beneficiary Cost Sharing Liability Under Medicare as a Percent
       of Median Income for Elderly   40
3.1   Per Enrollee HI Benefit Payments Adjusted by Alternative Price
       Deflators, 1975–95   48
3.2   Per Enrollee SMI Benefit Payments Adjusted by Alternative Price
       Deflators, 1975–95   50
3.3   Annual Rates of Growth in Medicare Hospital Payments,
       1975–93   54
3.4   Average Length of Stay in Nonfederal Short-Stay Hospitals,
       1980–93   61
3.5   Aggregate PPS Operating Margins   64
3.6   Estimated Balance in Federal Hospital Insurance Trust Fund,
       Selected Years, 1982–2003   67
3.7   Annual Rates of Growth in Medicare Physician Payments,
       1976–93   70
3.8   Benefit Payments Under Medicare Part A: 1975–93   80
4.1   Per Capita Medicare Expenditures: Federal Share and
       Beneficiary Liability, Adjusted for Inflation   90
4.2   Assignment Rates for Part B Claims for Medicare, CY 1969–94   95
4.3   Average Length of Stay in Nonfederal Short-Stay Hospitals, by
       Age, 1980–93   101
5.1   Additional Premiums Under Selected Catastrophic Plans by
       Adjusted Gross Income, 1989   122
7.1   Medicare Spending by All Elderly by Age, 1986   191
7.2   Medicare Spending by Decedents by Age, 1985   191

FOREWORD

When the first edition of *Medicare Now and in the Future* was published, many were predicting that reform of Medicare would be part of a comprehensive restructuring of the nation's healthcare system—public and private. For that reason, one of Marilyn Moon's major goals in her previous book was to help readers focus on Medicare in the context of broader health system reform. Three years later, such comprehensive reform no longer appears imminent.

As interest in system reform has waned, however, the focus on reforming Medicare has increased, simply because, in a political climate of budget balancing and government downsizing, its size makes it a major candidate for cuts. Moon takes the occasion of the 30th anniversary of Medicare's first beneficiary payment to take another hard look at the program. Recognizing the constraints imposed by the current budget climate and an aging population, she discusses how the Medicare budget can be tightened, and providers and beneficiaries made more cost-conscious in their use of care, without threatening the well-being of elderly and disabled Americans—two vulnerable populations whose major source of acute care is the Medicare program.

Her fundamental point is that better targeting can lead to budget savings without threatening quality of care. Large cuts are possible in some areas, in her judgment, if they are combined with selective increases in others. Across-the-board cuts are never the right answer.

A major focus of Moon's new book is the issue of means-testing—making better-off beneficiaries pay more for their care. As is true for the rest of the population, the gap between rich and poor among the elderly is growing. The Medicare trust fund faces bankruptcy by the year 2001 and the proportion of the nonelderly without insurance protection, particularly children, is rising. These are times when it is essential to revisit the original premise of the Medicare program that elderly and disabled Americans should be entitled to healthcare protection without regard to income differences. Moon provides a detailed analysis of the kinds of increased financial burdens the elderly can reasonably be expected to bear and those they cannot.

Because reform of the Medicare program—which now accounts for over 10 percent of the federal budget—will almost inevitably be a prominent part of the budget debate for years to come, the issues discussed in this book are important in a policy arena that stretches beyond healthcare reform. It is my hope that Moon's considered treatment of them will illuminate what is often a heated rather than enlightening debate.

William Gorham
President
July, 1996

PREFACE TO THE SECOND EDITION

The first edition of this monograph fulfilled a long-term ambition of mine to write in depth about the Medicare program. I have been working on Medicare issues since 1981 and found that there was little in the literature that described the program or recognized its complexities—issues that are crucial to a reasonable debate over changes that need to be made over time. And although there has been little in the way of substantive legislative change in the Medicare program since 1992 when most of the work on the first edition was underway, a number of factors have now dated this edition. The rate of growth of spending on Medicare, for example, has been such that the numbers from the first edition are now out of date.

And even more important is the changing context of the healthcare environment of which Medicare is a part. Enthusiasm for healthcare reform for the younger population was very strong; in fact, some advocates of reform even suggested using the Medicare program as the basis for systemwide reforms. Times have changed substantially in just four short years, however. Suspicion of government programs is high—although Medicare remains popular. And both sides of the political aisle now talk about reducing the size of government overall. Further, the Medicare program is insufficiently financed for the near term and will later face even greater challenges from the aging of our population.

Consequently, what at first was a plan to update the numbers and modestly rewrite several of the last chapters of this book evolved into a major effort to recast the book in the context of the current policy discussion. Chapters 1, 6, 7, and 9 have been largely rewritten. Some options, such as combining changes in Medicare with broader reforms, are not on the agenda at present. In addition, options for reform such as vouchers—which constituted esoteric discussions in 1992—are now getting serious attention. The introduction and policy chapters have thus been reworked to accommodate such changes. The basic structure of the book remains much the same, however. The history of the program contained in chapters 2 through 5 has only been modestly updated. Finally, I did little to revise chapter 8, which considers possible expansions of Medicare. The problems that prompted proposed expansions have not diminished—only the likelihood of addressing them in the near term has. Thus, I have retained that chapter here, even though it is not of as much current interest as it would have been just two or three years ago.

Many colleagues read and critiqued the first edition. I remain indebted to them. In particular, John Holahan and Judith Feder devoted considerable effort to helping me with the original manuscript.

And since its original publication, I have had many spirited discussions with colleagues at the Institute over various aspects of Medicare, including Stephen Zuckerman, Genevieve Kenney, Margaret Sulvetta, and Korbin Liu. A recent joint paper on options for Medicare savings with these colleagues is frequently cited herein and affected my views in a number of areas. A recent article I co-authored with Karen Davis also helped with my rethinking of issues. Robert Myers noted a number of errors in the first edition, which I endeavored to correct in this version. Judy Feder and John Holahan also continue to play important roles as thoughtful critics; I appreciate their generosity with their time and their support of my work.

Crystal Kuntz helped in many ways with the revisions. She produced tables, tracked down data, oversaw revision of the references, and carefully read the manuscript. Laurie Pounder also provided valuable research assistance. Felicity Skidmore, on a very tight time schedule, did her usual skillful job of clarifying and improving the manuscript.

Finally, I am most indebted to Douglas Gomery, whose dedication to his own work and professionalism sets a standard I seldom meet. But I keep trying. Even so, he continues to be my biggest fan and I am deeply grateful for his support.

The first edition of this book was largely financed by general support from the Urban Institute. In addition, a grant from the Retirement Research Foundation provided some additional funding. For the second edition, some of the new data in the options chapters are based on earlier work funded by the Henry J. Kaiser Family Foundation. But most of the new work was made possible by support from the Commonwealth Fund's program on Medicare's Future. I hope this book will serve as an anchor for further work in Medicare now underway at the Institute thanks to the Commonwealth Fund.

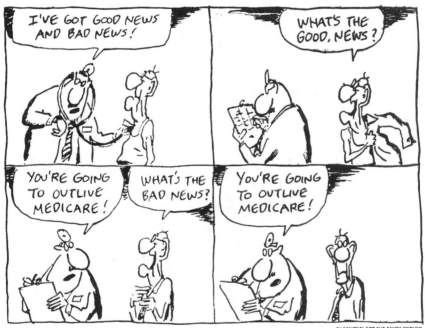

Chapter One

PLACING MEDICARE IN CONTEXT

Medicare has contributed substantially to the well-being of America's oldest and most disabled citizens. It is the largest public healthcare program in the United States, providing the major source of insurance for acute care for the elderly and disabled populations. For some, Medicare represents a model of what national health insurance could be in the United States. Its administrative costs are low, and it is popular with both its beneficiaries and the general population. At the same time, Medicare is one of the fastest growing programs in the federal budget, gobbling up new resources at the rate of 15 percent each year during its first 30 years. Critics assail the program as being out of sync with the needs of many senior citizens through its failure to provide long-term care coverage. It is the subject of endless criticism and debate by physicians and hospital administrators, who nonetheless rely upon it for a substantial share of their revenues. Some proponents of change would fully privatize the program, but most proposals to privatize Medicare would retain the current program as a fallback.

In 1995, Medicare consumed $177 billion in federal outlays. Nearly every year since 1980, it has been a major focus of budget reduction efforts. And in 1995, projected seven-year savings of $226 billion made it the largest component of savings in the Balanced Budget Act, which was vetoed by President Clinton. The controversy over the appropriate size and funding for the program will continue for the foreseeable future as the pressures on financing the program grow. This book examines the current status of Medicare and offers options for reform with a particular focus on the program's beneficiaries: What is Medicare, how does it work, and where is it headed? What are the problems facing Medicare, and how can they be resolved? What options for the future hold the most promise?

WHY EXAMINE MEDICARE NOW?

The portion of the federal budget devoted to healthcare has been expanding rapidly since 1965, when Medicare was introduced as a program to meet the healthcare needs of aged Americans. Critics pointed out early on that Medicare spending was likely to grow rapidly; and grow it did. For example, in 1970, spending on Medicare totaled $6.8 billion, about 3.5 percent of the total federal budget. Twenty years later, that share had more than doubled as Medicare accounted for 8.6 percent of the federal budget and about $107 billion in outlays (U.S. Congress, House Committee on Ways and Means [henceforth, Ways and Means] 1991) (see figure 1.1). By 1995, the share had grown to 10.5 percent of the budget (Office of the President 1996).

This rapid increase is outstripping the growth in dedicated revenues to support the hospital portion of Medicare. In 1995, payments out of the program exceeded revenues coming in, signaling the inevitable exhaustion of the Federal Hospital Insurance Trust Fund if no policy changes are made.[1] After postponing the date of reckoning consistently for years—by undertaking various cost-cutting efforts and increasing the wage base subject to taxation—the latest Medicare trustees report predicts the date of exhaustion to be 2001 (Board of Trustees, Federal Hospital Insurance Trust Fund [henceforth, HI Trustees] 1996). The trustees' report for 1996, as it has for several years, indicates that the fund does not meet the short-run test for solvency.

Because of its size and rapid growth, Medicare also became a target of budget reduction efforts, beginning in earnest with the administration of Ronald Reagan. Every budget submission by Presidents Reagan and George Bush contained proposals for substantial cuts in Medicare. Many of those cost-containment changes, particularly in the area of provider reimbursement, were enacted by the U.S. Congress in the 1980s. The budget reduction efforts of President Clinton in 1993 cut Medicare spending by $56 billion over a five-year period. Budget stalemate in 1995 precluded further changes. But both sides of the political aisle agree that more spending reductions will be needed since Medicare has continued to expand. Any legislative cuts have been more than outweighed by spending growth. In Medicare, "cuts" of even billions of dollars do not mean declines in spending—just a slower rate of increase (see figure 1.2).

Because Medicare is such a large component of the federal budget, it receives particular scrutiny for further sources of budget reductions. Further, most of its enrollees are over age 65, and in the last several

Figure 1.1 MEDICARE AS SHARE OF FEDERAL BUDGET, 1965–95

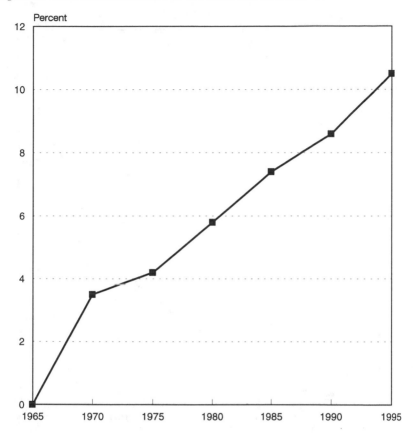

Source: U.S. Congress, House Committee on Ways and Means (henceforth, Ways and Means) (1994); Office of the President (1996).

years, the growing share of the budget devoted to older Americans has been noted with alarm by conservatives and liberals alike. Some claim that more resources should be freed up for children, others that too much public money is spent on the elderly.

At the same time that much of the focus in Medicare has been on reducing spending, critics argue that the program inadequately meets the needs of the aged and disabled. Medicare's coverage is less generous than that offered many younger families and individuals through employer-subsidized insurance. The ill-fated Medicare Catastrophic Coverage Act of 1988 sought to fill in some of those gaps, but that legislation was repealed just 18 months after passage. The failed

Figure 1.2 ANNUAL FEDERAL OUTLAYS FOR MEDICARE, 1967–2000

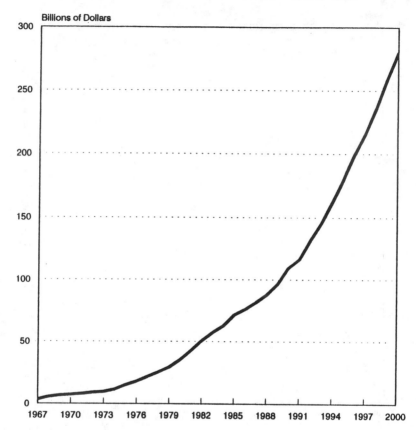

Source: Office of the President (1996).

attempts to enact comprehensive healthcare reforms in the early 1990s would not have expanded Medicare, but did propose a modest program to meet some of the long-term care needs of elderly and disabled persons. Although this would have been a separate program, supporters of expanded long-term care benefits often seek to add such coverage to Medicare.[2]

In many ways, Medicare was of only secondary concern in the debate over broader reform from 1992 to 1994. Medicare would have largely been kept separate from other reforms, and was treated as "untouchable" even by those advocating sweeping changes elsewhere (Moon 1994). Less popular approaches would have folded Medicare into a fully public system, or "privatized" it to conform to a similar market-based reform plan for younger families. But while the collapse of general health reform proposals in the first half of the 1990s has meant little discussion about change for the general population, interest in Medicare has actually increased. But the new concern stems more from discussions about downsizing government than from interest in Medicare per se.

Four areas of pressure will shape the future of Medicare. First, Medicare was established to help the elderly, and then disabled persons, to afford medical care. Thus, the economic status of these two groups—and particularly the elderly—is a critical factor in assessing how the system ought to change. Second, what happens in the healthcare system overall clearly affects Medicare. In many ways, the problems facing Medicare are but a reflection of the broader problems facing healthcare in the United States. Most observers agree that at least some of the solutions to Medicare's problems should apply systemwide, although systemwide reform efforts seem less likely than just a few years ago. Third, Medicare's future as a public program is tied to the financing problems facing the federal government during a period of fiscal restraint. So long as budget deficits continue at the federal level, changes in Medicare will be caught up in the pressure to limit all types of federal spending. Finally, the demographic changes looming on the horizon—which will swell the ranks of those eligible for benefits and diminish the number of workers financing the system—are beginning to influence the debate even about Medicare's near-term future.

ECONOMIC STATUS OF OLDER AMERICANS

By every measure of economic well-being, the situation for older Americans has improved substantially over the past three decades. For example, incomes for those 65 and older have risen steadily, from a median per capita income of $3,408 in 1975 to $10,808 in 1993 (U.S. Bureau of the Census 1991 and 1996). After controlling for inflation, this represents a gain of 18 percent in the purchasing power of this age group. Moreover, in the 1980s, the elderly's income growth outstripped increases in income for younger subgroups of the population. Although average before-tax incomes for elderly families still lag behind those of younger families, after adjusting for differences in family size and tax liabilities, the disposable (posttax) per capita incomes of older Americans do not differ substantially from those of their younger counterparts (Danziger et al. 1984; Smeeding 1986). Income growth in the 1990s seems to be proceeding similarly for both the young and the old.

But to fully comprehend the ability of elderly individuals to meet their needs, it is crucial to look beyond averages and to understand the diversity of the resources available to this group. Although the elderly have shown impressive gains as a group, not every elderly individual has shared in the good fortune. For example, some of the increase in well-being associated with comparisons of incomes across time reflects the changing composition of the elderly. Each year individuals turning age 65 join the elderly "category," and the incomes of new cohorts of 65-year-olds tend, on average, to be higher each year. As a result, individuals within the elderly population display much slower rates of income growth than does the group as a whole. For example, as shown in table 1.1, growth in median incomes for all persons 65 and over averaged 7.1 percent for men and 4.9 percent for women between 1985 and 1990 (after controlling for inflation). But if, instead, we followed the cohort of persons aged 65 to 69 in 1985 (who were 70 to 74 in 1990), incomes rose much more slowly and actually declined for men.

On a more positive note, elderly poverty has declined. The share of the elderly in poverty dropped from 25 percent in 1968 to 11.7 percent in 1994 (U.S. Bureau of the Census 1995a). In 1982, for the first time, the official rate of poverty among the elderly was lower than that for the rest of the population. The largest declines in poverty rates for the elderly occurred before 1975, however, and the rates have remained relatively flat since 1984 (see figure 1.3).

It should also be noted that the Census figures may understate poverty rates for the elderly relative to other groups. First, the traditional poverty thresholds presented for older persons are deliberately set

Table 1.1 GROWTH IN MEDIAN INCOME FOR ALL ELDERLY AND FOR SPECIFIC COHORT IN THE UNITED STATES, 1985–90

	Median Income, 1990 ($)	Real Income Growth, 1985–90 (%)
Men		
All 65 and older	14,183	7.1
Aged 65–69 in 1985	14,665	−4.1
Women		
All 65 and older	8,044	4.9
Aged 65–69 in 1985	8,160	2.9

Source: U.S. Bureau of the Census (1986, 1991).

Figure 1.3 POVERTY RATES IN THE UNITED STATES FOR PERSONS AGED 65
AND OLDER, 1966–94

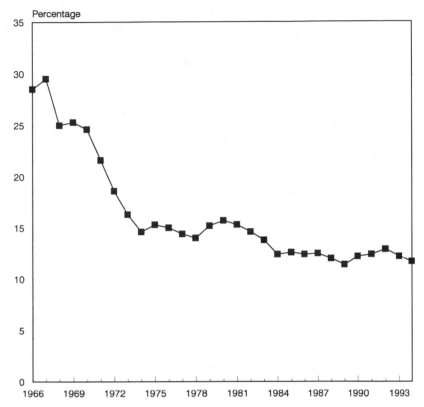

Source: U.S. Bureau of the Census (1995a).

lower than those for younger families. There is little evidence today
to justify such a differentiation. Applying the same poverty threshold
for the elderly as is used for other groups would increase the poverty
rates for older Americans from 12.4 to 15.4 percent (1992 data). Even
these thresholds may be too low, since adjustments have only been
made for inflation, not for changes in general expectations concerning
living standards (Ruggles 1990).

Second, and more important, if the burdens of high out-of-pocket
healthcare spending were taken into account, elderly poverty rates
would rise even further. Although Medicare, Medicaid, and employer-
subsidized insurance reduce the burdens on older Americans, this
group still faces much higher unreimbursed spending on health services compared to other families. The standard poverty thresholds

now in use do not account for this additional burden (National Resource Council 1995). Adding the average out-of-pocket spending to the standard poverty thresholds would yield a poverty rate for elderly persons of over 20 percent in 1992 (Moon and Mulvey 1996).[3]

The share of the elderly in poverty is also sensitive to the large number of older persons now clustered just above the official poverty line. In 1994, 3.7 million individuals 65 or older were listed as poor. Another 2.2 million have incomes of no more than 25 percent above the poverty threshold. When we count the total number with incomes below 150 percent of the poverty threshold, 26.3 percent of the elderly—about 8.2 million persons—had very limited incomes (U.S. Bureau of the Census 1995a).

It is true that the elderly do hold more assets, on average, than other families with low and moderate incomes. But even if assets were incorporated into poverty measures, only a small share of the poor would have their incomes boosted to any major degree (Moon and Mulvey 1996). Elderly families in the bottom one-fifth of all households have assets other than their homes averaging less than $4,000 (Bureau of the Census 1994b).

Finally, when evaluating the well-being of the elderly, it is important to remember that income inequality has been widening for all age groups ever since the late 1970s. Incomes for the low-income elderly have been growing, but they have been growing at consistently lower rates than incomes for the high-income elderly (Ways and Means 1994).

What about elderly persons with substantial resources? This is the group that many policymakers would target for cuts in Medicare benefits. As table 1.2 indicates, the top 20 percent of elderly couples had incomes averaging $75,062 in 1992, and the highest one-fifth of singles averaged $32,588. The next highest quintile had an average in-

Table 1.2 AVERAGE FAMILY INCOME OF OLDER AMERICANS BY QUINTILE, 1992

Quintile[a]	Singles ($)	Couples ($)	All Elderly Families
First	4,301	9,607	6,272
Second	7,267	17,608	12,493
Third	10,342	24,953	19,607
Fourth	15,051	35,047	30,186
Highest	32,588	75,062	66,829
All	13,900	47,842	40,238

Source: Current Population Survey, U.S. Bureau of the Census, March 1993.
a. Quintiles provide a ranking of income from high to low, with each quintile representing one-fifth of the total individuals or families in the comparison.

come substantially below that of the highest quintile, dropping by more than half in each case.

In sum, the dichotomy between the wealthiest and the poorest older Americans is growing, creating new challenges for public policy. Should the highest-income elderly, for example, contribute substantially more to their care? The answer hinges on society's judgment on a whole variety of issues, but one important one is how well off we perceive them to be relative to younger Americans at the top of the distribution. Making such a comparison is difficult and controversial, because families at different ages have such different sizes, needs, and opportunities.

Prospects for the Future

If the trends of the last decade were taken as projections into the next, we would expect to see continued steady growth in average incomes of the elderly, continued improvement relative to the working population, and a general trend toward lower poverty rates. Evidence from the 1950–80 Censuses (Ross, Danziger, and Smolensky 1987) and from wealth surveys taken between 1962 and 1983 (Wolff 1987) indicates that the next generation of elderly—that is, those born between 1920 and 1935, and reaching age 65 between 1985 and 2000—will be considerably better off as they age than their older counterparts. This group had the good fortune to be in their prime working years during the period of maximum earnings growth of the halcyon 1960s, to find the value of their homes soaring during the inflation of the 1970s, and to be in the maximum liquid asset position to capture most fully the benefits of high real interest rates and the stock market boom of the early to mid-1980s.

But projecting past trends almost certainly paints too rosy a picture. There are several reasons for caution in assuming ever-rising increases in economic status for the elderly. The rate of growth of Social Security benefits has already slackened, and the slow growth in average wages for current workers will limit their benefits as retirees. Income from private pensions, which has shown rapid growth in recent years, now seems to be leveling off. And the proportion of the population receiving pensions will not grow as rapidly in the future.

The changing age composition of the elderly will also retard the extent to which incomes grow over time. The very old will increase as a proportion of the elderly, and their lower average incomes are likely to help hold down overall rates of growth in income as compared to the growth of the 1970s. The younger old will be better off, but the over-85 age group will constitute an increasing share of the elderly population. In the near future, as the elderly population grows more as a result of longer life spans than because of new "entrants" to the 65 and over category, income growth will tend to be slower. In the 1990s, growth in the numbers of persons 65 and over will be concentrated in the over age-85 category, reflecting increased life expectancies. Individuals reaching retirement age will have been born in the 1930s, a period when birth rates were very low. Between 1990 and the year 2000, the population between the ages of 65 and 74 will grow by only 1.2 percent, while the group of those aged 85 and above will grow by 34 percent (Ways and Means 1992).

If these moderating influences on growth hold and the economy experiences relatively rapid real growth in the next decade, the status of the elderly relative to the young could again decline. More likely, however, the economic position of the elderly will stabilize relative to their younger counterparts. Growth in incomes for both the elderly and the young will likely average out to a moderate pace over the near term. This *relative* status of the elderly—both the high- and the low-income elderly—is likely to be important in any political debates over who should pay for Medicare, since many of the potential policy alternatives involve trade-offs between burdens on the old and burdens on the young.

Burdens from Health Spending

The percentage of income spent on healthcare by persons over age 65 is at an all-time high and will increase further. This spending now represents a critical burden for the elderly, averaging about 21 percent of the incomes of typical elderly persons in 1994. For certain groups of the population, the share is even higher (see Table 1.3). These figures have risen steadily over the years and are up from 15 percent in 1987 (AARP 1995). Preliminary estimates indicate the share spent on acute healthcare services by older Americans will rise to about 23 percent for 1996. Incomes have risen rapidly for this age group, but out-of-pocket health costs have simply risen faster.[4]

While most elderly persons now have supplemental coverage to help pay for health costs (see figure 1.4), that does not necessarily reduce the burden of paying for that care. The purchase of private supplemental coverage, often termed "Medigap," is not a solution, since it tends to *raise* the average spending on healthcare. Since many older Americans pay fully for this insurance, they are effectively still bearing the burden of healthcare costs, plus paying an additional amount

Table 1.3 HEALTH CARE SPENDING OUT-OF-POCKET AND ON PREMIUMS AS SHARE OF INCOME

	Percentage of Elderly	Per Capita Spending ($)		Health Expenditure as Share of Family Income (%)[a]
		Out-of-Pocket	Insurance Premiums	
Poverty Status:				
Under 100%	12.1	913	653	34
100–125%	8.0	1,047	1,069	27
125–200%	20.5	1,456	1,268	26
200–400%	35.1	1,486	1,200	18
Over 400%	24.4	1,509	1,199	13
Age:				
65–69	33.7	972	1,078	18
70–74	26.5	1,121	1,143	19
75–79	19.9	1,357	1,231	20
80–84	11.5	2,296	1,193	31
85 +	8.4	2,700	1,082	29
Total	—	1,382	1,137	21

Source: Moon and Mulvey (1995).
a. Although the dollars shown in this table are per capita, the shares of income are estimated by family, recognizing that it is family budgets and combined spending that matter.

Figure 1.4 HEALTH INSURANCE SUPPLEMENTING MEDICARE: 1991

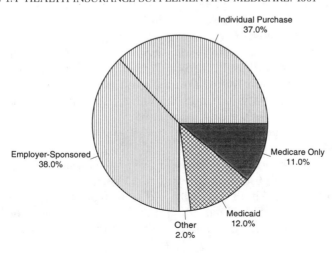

Source: Chulis et al. (1993).

to cover the often substantial administrative costs of the insurance (Feder et al. 1987a). Because so many older persons have relatively high expenditures, this insurance does not spread the risks of health spending enough to result in lower costs for the average individual. Medigap does help reduce the chances of high burdens in any one year, but does not address the basic problem of affordability.

Two major areas of protection are available for the elderly, one at each end of the income distribution. At the bottom, Medicaid fills in the gaps through either its traditional benefits for low-income persons or the newer Qualified Medicare Beneficiary and Specified Low Income Beneficiary programs.[5] At the higher end of the distribution, about 38 percent of older persons have supplemental coverage from a former employer (Chulis et al. 1993). Although this employer coverage is usually only for acute care, it does offer important relief for those who have it since premium costs are usually subsidized.[6]

The costs of long-term care hold the potential for even more devastating reductions in economic status for older families. The burdens imposed by these costs are hard to evaluate in general, but on a case-by-case basis, an individual pays, on average, more than $35,000 for a year's stay in a nursing home. Medicare pays for only a small share of long-term care, and Medicaid will only cover these costs once an individual has spent down nearly all of his or her assets. Even with the expanded Medicaid protection to lessen the impact of this "spend down" that was established by the Medicare Catastrophic Coverage Act, the spouse remaining in the community often faces a much-reduced standard of living. It is under these conditions that even middle-class elderly families find it financially impossible to meet their healthcare needs.

The likelihood of incurring costs from both acute and long-term healthcare rises steadily with age—in reverse proportion to ability to pay. An elderly woman living alone is most at risk of needing long-term care services (Doty, Liu, and Wiener 1985). And the outlook for the future is not reassuring. Wiener et al. (1994) suggest that only a minority of older families will ever be able to afford long-term care expenditures.

The burdens of healthcare will expand faster than the elderly's ability to pay for the foreseeable future. Over the same period that median incomes rose 18 percent, real out-of-pocket spending on healthcare more than doubled. To conclude that we have solved the financial challenges facing older Americans is therefore premature.

THE ECONOMIC STATUS OF DISABLED PERSONS

Medicare is usually seen as a program for the over-65 population, but it covers younger disabled Americans as well. Relatively little is known about the economic status of the over 4 million disabled Medicare beneficiaries, who constitute about 12 percent of all Medicare beneficiaries. By definition, such individuals must be unable to work, so unless other family members are in the labor force, the family is likely to face severe economic constraints. Moreover, the onset of disability may occur in conjunction with high levels of spending on medical care and high rates of absenteeism from the workplace. Both of these factors may serve as a drain on the resources of the disabled worker and of his or her family. Disabled persons must then wait for two years after qualifying for Social Security benefits to become eligible for benefits.

One recent study found that disabled Social Security recipients were more likely to be poor in comparison to either the general population or persons receiving Social Security as retired workers (Grad 1989).[7] The rate of poverty was 19 percent for these disabled persons, and an additional 11 percent were near poor. By comparison, only 17 percent of retired workers were poor or near poor. Moreover, disabled workers are even less likely to have assets upon which to draw than are their older counterparts, since the former have not had as many years or opportunities to accumulate wealth.

Thus, although details on the economic status of Medicare disabled beneficiaries are sketchy, this group has much in common with older beneficiaries. Like the elderly, a disproportionate number are poor, and there is a considerable disparity between the rich and poor among them. Moreover, out-of-pocket healthcare costs are likely to represent a considerable burden on this group, since their average Medicare expenditures are higher even than for the elderly.[8] And they are less likely to have supplemental insurance. Since they are not retirees, they are unlikely to have employer-sponsored benefits, and traditional Medigap policies are not offered to this population group.

THE PROBLEM OF RISING HEALTHCARE COSTS

The problems driving Medicare costs upward are not unique to the public sector. They are found throughout our nation's healthcare system, and the crisis of rising healthcare costs affects all payers: individuals, businesses, and governments. Although Medicare has been a leader in experimenting with options for curbing the costs of care, both in terms of increasing prices and use of services, costs continue to rise.

Prices

During the 1970s healthcare prices rose rapidly, but at about the same rate as all prices in the economy. In the 1980s, however, the general rise in consumer prices slowed, whereas growth in healthcare prices remained high. As figure 1.5 indicates, prices followed essentially the same track until 1975, when rates of increase began to diverge. After 1980, inflation in the price of healthcare occurred at rates substantially higher than that for the overall index. Since then, the medical care component of the consumer price index (CPI) has never been below the rate of growth of the remaining components. Between 1980 and 1990, all consumer prices grew 58.6 percent, whereas the CPI for healthcare grew 117.4 percent (Office of the President 1992b). Only in the last few years have medical care prices begun to moderate relative to the CPI as a whole.

What caused this inflation in healthcare prices during a decade when the rate of growth of other prices slowed substantially? Some economists point to the fact that healthcare is heavily service oriented, with rising wages in these areas translating directly into rising prices. It is difficult to find ways to cut costs per service. Productivity thus does not rise much in this sector of the economy. Yet, costs of manufactured goods like pharmaceuticals are also increasing faster than inflation in general.

Nor is it possible to blame the inflation in healthcare prices on strong demand for scarce services. The supply of physicians continued its rapid growth through both the 1970s and 1980s. For example, in 1970 the number of active physicians per 10,000 population stood at 15.6. By 1988, the number was 23.3 (National Center for Health Statistics [henceforth, NCHS] 1991). This greater supply of physicians did not, however, lower their incomes, which rose an average of 8.6 percent per year from 1979 to 1988 (see figure 1.6). Further, hospitals operated at much less than capacity throughout the 1980s, with occupancy rates averaging about 64 percent in 1993 (American Hospital Association [henceforth, AHA] 1995).

Much of the explanation for rising prices undoubtedly rests with the fact that until very recently the price structure of the healthcare

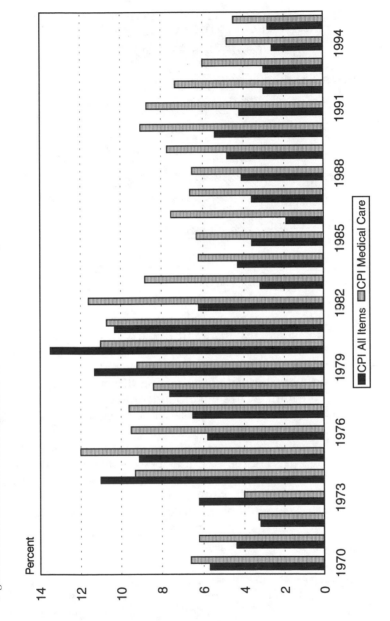

Figure 1.5 HEALTHCARE PRICE INFLATION IN THE UNITED STATES, 1970–1995

Source: Bureau of Labor Statistics (1996).

Figure 1.6 AVERAGE ANNUAL GROWTH RATES IN PHYSICIAN NET INCOME BY SPECIALTY IN THE UNITED STATES, 1979–88

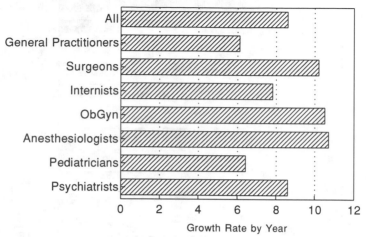

Source: American Medical Association, 1988.

industry had not come under heavy scrutiny. Users of healthcare are typically not the payers; usually a "third party" such as an insurance company or the government pays for the care. Insured people do not choose who to see or what to use on the basis of the prices charged. Moreover, even when the patient is paying directly, people facing a medical crisis are unlikely to shop around for the least expensive care or to question the need for various services. In short, the market for healthcare goods and services does not foster price competition. Recent criticism leveled at the medical care price index also suggests that it, like other parts of the CPI, may be overstated (Huskamp and Newhouse 1994). Quality improvements and the degree of discounting that now exists are not well captured by this measure. Nonetheless, price inflation has certainly played a role in rapidly rising costs.

Use of Services

Despite price rises, the use of services has also continued to increase. This occurs not so much in terms of overall numbers of visits but in the type and complexity of healthcare services (often referred to as "intensity"). To some extent, this is related to new technology that has given us new tools such as computerized tomography (CT) scans and magnetic resonance imagers (MRIs), and new procedures such as endoscopies and arthroscopies. These new sources of healthcare spending tend to operate as additions to goods and services consumed, rather than as replacements for old technologies or procedures. For example, people may now receive x-rays, CT scans, and MRIs to diagnose a problem, whereas before only x-rays (and perhaps exploratory surgery) were available. As another example, rather than subjecting a blood sample to one test, it is now simple to run 30 or 40 tests per sample. The availability of new tests and procedures that are less invasive and painful has surely improved diagnosis and treatment for many Americans—and increased the frequency of their use. Some argue that these services are overused, when less advanced tests or fewer alternative tests would be sufficient. But for the average patient, there is little reason to resist using these tools. And, not only are physicians paid well for these extra tests, but the tests may reduce the time necessary to make a diagnosis.

These new procedures are not cheap. Medicare's average payment for an MRI of the brain, for example, which was not available at all in 1980, was $879 in 1993 (Zuckerman, Verrilli and Norton 1996). Similarly, the "scopes" also carry hefty price tags; for instance, Medicare paid $284 for a diagnostic colonoscopy in 1993, and private sector charges are even higher. New drugs to treat problems such as hypertension or blood clots after heart attacks can run into the thousands of dollars.

The number of physician contacts with specialists is also on the rise (NCHS 1991), and the supply of physicians reflects this trend. Between 1975 and 1993, the number of general and family practitioners increased only 25.3 percent, while the number of cardiovascular disease specialists grew by 139.7 percent, orthopedic surgeons by 100.2 percent, and gastroenterologists by 271.0 percent (NCHS 1995). These figures also indicate that use is shifting to higher cost services over time.

Surgery and other technical procedures continue to grow, albeit in different settings than in the past. The number of inpatient surgical operations fell by 4.6 percent between 1980 and 1989 (NCHS 1991), largely because of the enormous number of outpatient surgical procedures that now occur in a variety of settings. The American Hospital Association (AHA) has reported that 55.4 percent of total hospital-based surgeries are now performed in their outpatient departments, as compared to just 16.4 percent in 1980 (AHA 1994). And many procedures such as cataract surgery are now done in free-standing surgical centers or even physicians' offices.

The remaining inpatient surgeries are also becoming increasingly more complex and expensive. Across the 1980 to 1993 period, the rate of tonsillectomies dropped dramatically. Expensive procedures showed the opposite trend. For example, cardiac bypass surgery rates rose for men over the age of 75, from 0.9 per 1,000 in 1980 to 8.7 per 1,000 in 1993 (NCHS 1995).

The improved success of procedures such as hip replacements and cataract surgery means that outcomes have improved whereas the risks of surgeries have fallen.[9] In such cases, higher rates of use would certainly be expected and appropriate. The value of these procedures to individuals has increased over time. And lowered risks mean that older or disabled patients are particularly more likely to benefit now. It should not be surprising, then, that costs of care for these groups are rising rapidly. In fact, it is likely that some of the increase in use is a reflection of the greater value of such services, and of beneficiaries choosing to consume more of them.

The problem, of course, is in determining what proportion of the overall increase is desirable and what proportion might indicate excessive use. Cataract surgery offers a good example. We do not know what share of its explosive growth occurs because people with early cataracts are encouraged to obtain the operation before it is medically appropriate and what share reflects surgeries that truly improve the quality of life for patients.

These issues are not confined to Medicare; they are pervasive in the U.S. healthcare system. In fact, Medicare has been relatively successful in holding the line on costs in the 1980s, as compared with rates of growth in healthcare spending paid by private insurance. This comparison is proffered in figure 1.7, which shows annual rates of growth in per capita spending in Medicare and private insurance from the national health expenditure accounts on a selected set of services. These services—hospital care, physicians and other professional services, and vision and durable medical equipment—are those which are consistently covered by both Medicare and private insurance.[10] Between 1985 and 1992 Medicare had lower rates of growth—often considerably lower—than did private insurance.[11] While the picture in the last year or two will show the private sector holding down spending growth, a historical look at the data suggests that Medicare is not out of sync with the rest of the health care system. Indeed, the patterns in spending growth are very similar.

Medicare cannot be successful in holding down costs over the long run if healthcare spending in general is escalating. As stated, the pressures driving costs upward come from all parts of the healthcare system. Although Medicare commands a substantial share of the healthcare market, it cannot, by itself, fully control use or prices.

Figure 1.7 PER CAPITA GROWTH RATES OF SERVICES COVERED BY BOTH MEDICARE AND PRIVATE INSURANCE

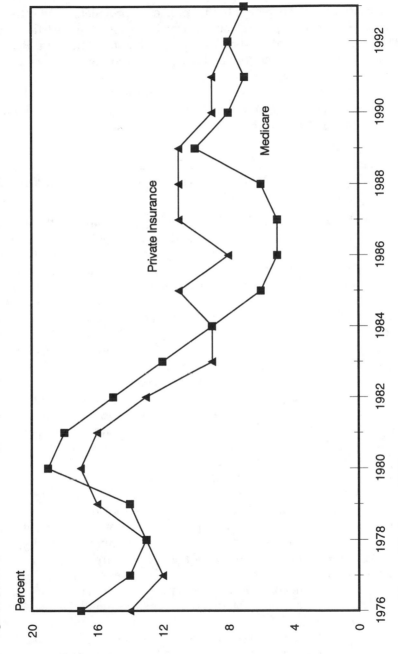

Source: Moon and Zuckerman (1995).

When Medicare acts alone, the response by providers can be to "divide and conquer," pitting one part of the system against the other. This constrains what Medicare can accomplish on its own. Broader system reform is needed for any long-run solution to Medicare's "cost problem." Expecting Medicare alone to carry this burden or to operate under a system unlike the rest of health care seems doomed to failure. But it is also unlikely that we will again take up the issue of broader reforms any time soon.

MEDICARE AS PART OF FEDERAL BUDGET

Although, relative to total healthcare costs, Medicare has done rather well in the 1980s, its absolute size and rate of growth cause Medicare to stand out from most other domestic programs in the federal budget. Since Medicare is funded by tax dollars in an era of antitax sentiment, it gets more scrutiny than health expenditures financed directly by individuals or businesses.[12] In the view of many policymakers, Medicare may be crowding out expenditures on other domestic programs and/or standing in the way of controlling the overall growth in federal expenditures. Such critics often argue that Americans will only accept a certain level of public spending, so if Medicare grows rapidly, it hurts other programs even if it has its own revenue source. This alone makes it a target.

Emphasis on balancing the federal budget—which dominated political debate in 1995—leads naturally to Medicare. The large share of the budget and the rapid growth rates in spending will likely keep it in the limelight for the foreseeable future.

Current law provides a fixed source of funding for the Hospital Insurance portion of Medicare—and the funding is not growing as fast as the level of spending, creating a potential future crisis when the trust fund becomes exhausted. The amount in this trust fund serves as an early warning of balance between financing and spending; its projected exhaustion is now about five years away. Even strong supporters of the Medicare program thus face the prospect that further changes will be needed in the next few years, either increasing the payroll tax rate devoted to Medicare or reexamining the generosity of the program itself.

In addition to budget pressures, Medicare is viewed with the same skepticism about government spending that affects Americans' perception of public programs generally. Because it is a government program, Medicare is automatically labeled bureaucratic and wasteful. In fact, evidence suggests that although Medicare is not without problems, in some cases these arise more from spending too little on administration rather than too much. For example, complaints about poor services and Medicare's complexity result in part from tight budgets for processing of claims. Compared to the private insurance sector, the Health Care Financing Administration's (HCFA) administrative costs for running the Medicare program are quite low, totaling only about 2 to 3 percent of benefit payments compared to larger proportional amounts—around 6 percent to 15 percent—for private insurers (Congressional Research Service [henceforth, CRS] 1989).

THE SPECIFIC FINANCING ISSUES FACING MEDICARE

Medicare faces its own financing challenges as well, particularly over the long run. Part A of the program (as described in the appendix) is financed by an earmarked set of revenues, principally a payroll tax. These revenues go into a trust fund that then pays out the benefits for that part of the program. For several years, this trust fund has been in financial difficulty, signaling an imbalance between revenues and expenditures. Indeed, when the 1995 trustees report was issued, again warning about the future insolvency of this trust fund, it became a political issue and lent support to congressional calls for major cuts in Medicare (Seib 1995).

This is a real problem, but not always exactly in the way it is described. First, both parts of the Medicare program are growing rapidly and at a faster pace than any source of revenue to pay for such spending. Part A is singled out because of the way its trust fund works, but the problem of high rates of growth in spending on Medicare is a problem facing the entire program.

Second, it has sometimes been implied that unless Medicare is cut, it will be necessary to stop paying benefits in a few years. There is not necessarily a cliff beyond which Medicare is unsalvageable. Indeed, the Part A trust fund has been within 10 years of exhaustion numerous times since 1970 (O'Sullivan 1995). Each time, modest changes have pushed back the date of exhaustion. Further, it is always possible to borrow from general revenues or other trust funds to keep the program going.[13] That is not to say such borrowing is good or desirable policy, but only that the trust fund imbalance should be viewed as a warning sign of major problems, not something unique or more serious than financing of other government programs.

Nonetheless, current projections put the date of trust fund exhaustion at 2001, just five years away (HI Trustees 1996). And even though we have been this close to exhaustion of the trust fund before, the rate of decline in the balance is projected to be more rapid than ever before. In 1995, income to and outflow from the Part A trust fund was essentially in balance with just a $35 million shortfall. But future income growth will average only 5.3 percent per year while outflows will average 8.6 percent, and be even higher in the near term (HI Trustees 1996). Such a discrepancy quickly draws down the balance and then erodes interest income as well. For example, if a deficit were allowed to accumulate in the Part A trust fund, it would total over $120 billion by the end of 2002 (see Figure 1.8).

The challenges are two. The first and more immediate challenge to Medicare is the danger of insolvency in the short run, which is driven by the high costs of health care. Since action in the near term will be needed, this issue is closely related to debates over the status of the current federal budget. The second is the demographic problem of the declining contributor-to-beneficiary ratio. The aging of the population will pose long-run challenges to the program and to the related Social Security program. Neither of these challenges has yet been addressed.

Most of the attention in the next few years will concentrate, appropriately, on reestablishing the solvency in the Part A trust fund for the next decade and slowing the rate of growth of spending on Part B. This will require attention to issues concerning the cost of health care and some debate over who should pay more to support the program. When the demographic issue is joined, a broader range of options will need to be considered, such as age of eligibility for Medicare.

RETHINKING MEDICARE POLICY

This volume has two main goals: to describe and analyze the growth and development of the Medicare program and to assess future options for change. Medicare rapidly enrolled first persons over 65 and then disabled individuals, offering them access to mainstream medical care. But in so doing, it led to a demand for more services that helped to create rapid growth in federal outlays. Much of Medicare's recent history has involved efforts to hold the line on cost growth. And although its growth has continued, Medicare has been relatively suc-

Figure 1.8 HI TRUST FUND ASSETS AT END OF THE YEAR, IN BILLIONS

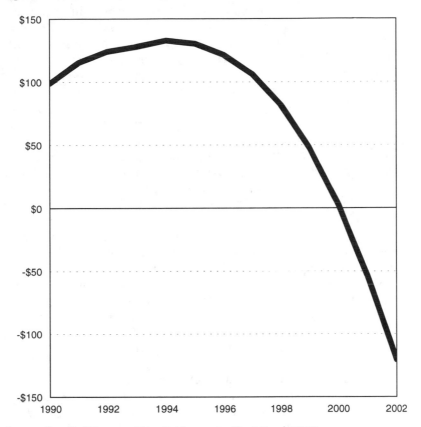

Source: Board of Trustees, Hospital Insurance Trust Fund (1996).

cessful at cost containment until very recently compared to the rest of the healthcare system, with innovations in hospital and physician payment that have led the way for the private sector.

But despite its successes, Medicare leaves many of its critics unsatisfied. Further reductions in spending will be sought by those concerned with the "bloated" size of the program, and some of those cuts are bound to occur in areas where we have already seen considerable change: payments to healthcare providers. Additional pressures will be levied on beneficiaries to pay more. Even in the absence of changes to save costs, Medicare cost sharing is due for reexamination. It is too high in some areas and too low in others and was never designed to influence incentives to consume healthcare services.

Some of the criticism calls for more substantive policy change. Incremental increases in premiums and cost sharing and in provider payments will not satisfy those who believe the program should be severely scaled back. In that case, more dramatic realignments would be needed. Calls for decentralizing the program and relying on the private sector to oversee a restructuring are also becoming increasingly popular. Counterbalancing these proposals are suggestions for expanding Medicare—adding better catastrophic protection, covering prescription drugs, or, most dramatically, bringing long-term care under Medicare's umbrella.

The first half of this book addresses the changes that Medicare has undergone and how well they have succeeded. Chapters 2, 3, and 4 divide Medicare's history into two general periods: first, an emphasis on access in the early years of the program, and then, beginning in the late 1970s, a shift to concern about cost containment. By the late 1980s, largely in response to cost-containment efforts, quality issues also became a secondary interest. Readers should note that the appendix at the end of this book will be of most interest to those unfamiliar with Medicare. The appendix defines basic components of the program (along with key terms) and can help put issues in context.

The second portion of this book begins with chapter 5's case study on a critical piece of legislation, the Medicare Catastrophic Coverage Act. The act's failure to elicit change in Medicare colors future policy for the program, strongly influencing how we get from here to "there." Chapter 6 considers possible marginal cost-containment measures as well as modest benefit expansions. Chapter 7 discusses broader options for reducing Medicare spending. Chapter 8 addresses the issues related to possible expansion of the system, although such plans are proffered less frequently in the mid-1990s.

Finally, chapter 9 concludes with my personal view of how Medicare should change and its relationship to general health system reform. Some changes could be instituted in the system regardless of the direction of health policy for the rest of the population. And indeed, reform in Medicare in the near term will likely be narrowly focused. But over time, change should be coordinated carefully, with policies adopted for the rest of our healthcare system either directly by government or indirectly as the marketplace dictates.

Notes

1. Hospital Insurance (Part A) covers hospital care, skilled nursing care, and home health benefits. Supplementary Medical Insurance (Part B) covers physician and other

ambulatory services. The two parts of the program are defined in more detail in the Appendix at the end of this book.

2. The distinction between acute care and long-term care is never absolute. Acute care refers to services, particularly in short-stay hospitals and physician services, that are used to treat a particular medical condition. Long-term care usually refers to supportive services for persons with chronic disabling conditions.

3. This is different from the approach sometimes taken to incorporating health spending in poverty measures, which adds in the value of Medicare and Medicaid to the resources a family has at its disposal (Smeeding 1984; Hurd 1989). Such an effort appears to lower the rates of poverty, but is distorted because it fails to take into account higher health care expenditures by the elderly. The way to deal comprehensively with this issue is to add Medicare and Medicaid to resources of the elderly, but also to add to the poverty threshold all health care spending. If done appropriately, this produces essentially the same result as simply adding out-of-pocket spending to the threshold measure (Moon and Mulvey 1996).

4. Some have suggested that this situation simply reflects that healthcare is a "luxury" good and that as incomes rise, we should expect to see more healthcare consumed. Some of this phenomenon may indeed be occurring, but as is discussed later, much of the rise in spending goes beyond simple increases in use of services.

5. These new programs are discussed in more detail in the appendix and in Chapters 2, 5 and 8. They were added to help ease the burdens of high cost sharing and premiums under Medicare for those with low incomes.

6. Moreover, the future of retiree coverage is somewhat uncertain as employers find the costs of covering existing employees burdensome. Anecdotal evidence suggests that there is beginning to be retrenchment in this area.

7. Disabled workers in this study are those receiving Social Security disability benefits. Since there is a two-year waiting period before such individuals become eligible for Medicare, they do not represent exactly the same population. The characteristics of these two overlapping groups are likely to be very similar, however.

8. Disabled persons and the elderly are combined in this analysis, unless otherwise noted.

9. As these various procedures have become more routine and less complicated to perform, it might be reasonable to expect facility and physician charges to fall—a phenomenon that largely does not occur. To at least some extent, this is related to the lack of a freely operating market for services.

10. But even if all health services were included in this figure, the basic pattern would look very much the same. High rates of growth in home health and nursing care under Medicare are somewhat offset by high rates of growth in prescription drugs that Medicare does not cover. The one exception would be 1989, when legislation expanded skilled nursing services under Medicare and a one-year spike in the rate of growth occurred that would cause Medicare to exceed private insurance in that year.

11. That Medicare's share of total health spending has been falling since 1985 is an especially important point, since there is often a misconception that the aging of the population must be a major factor in Medicare's growth. The number of beneficiaries is rising, but only at about 1.9 percent per year since 1982 (Committee on Ways and Means 1994).

12. Part A of Medicare is financed from earmarked payroll taxes—a mechanism that has largely protected Social Security from scrutiny. But interestingly, this has not insulated Medicare.

13. Social Security borrowed from Medicare's trust fund in the 1980s to get through a shortfall period until reforms in Social Security improved its financial situation, for example.

Chapter Two

ASSURING ACCESS

At its passage on July 28, 1965, the overriding goal of the Medicare program was to assure access to mainstream healthcare for persons over age 65. The elderly were underserved by the health system, largely because many older persons could not afford to obtain care. Insurance coverage as a part of retirement benefits was the exception and not the rule, and private insurance companies had shown a reluctance to offer coverage to older persons even when they could afford it.

In the early 1960s, older Americans were also disproportionately poor compared to the rest of the population. The 1962 poverty rate for elderly families was 47 percent, as opposed to 13 percent for families headed by someone aged 25 to 54 (Council of Economic Advisors 1964). Moreover, many more older persons had incomes just above the official poverty level of income. Health insurance was not as expensive then as today, but these very low-income individuals could not afford even modest insurance.

Some public support for low-income older Americans was available, primarily in the form of Medical Assistance to the Aged (MAA). This legislation was originally part of the Kerr-Mills bill, passed in 1960.[1] MAA required a means test, but it was not restricted to persons receiving public assistance. Rather, it was a federal/state matching program and depended on the willingness of states to set eligibility limits.[2] Although MAA can be viewed as a precursor of Medicare and Medicaid, it remained a very small program. In 1963, only 148,000 elderly persons received MAA, compared to Medicare's enrollment of 19 million persons by 1967 (Newman 1972). In 1965, MAA provided $523 million in medical benefits to the elderly, compared to Medicare spending in 1968 of $4.4 billion. In its first two years of existence, Medicare spending on the elderly poor grew to $2.1 billion—a fourfold increase (Plotnick and Skidmore 1975).

For higher-income elderly persons, the story was mixed. About half of all seniors had health insurance (Davis and Schoen 1978; Andersen et al. 1976). Generally, coverage could be obtained through former employers and from groups such as the American Association of Retired Persons (AARP). Indeed, health insurance was not merely an issue of affordability; it was also one of availability at any price. Private insurers had shown a reluctance to cover the elderly. Thus, although many of the elderly were needy with regard to healthcare, even in 1965 this was not a homogeneous group.

In contrast, coverage of workers through their employers was becoming increasingly common, underscoring the discrepancies between the elderly and nonelderly in access to care. Although health insurance was a relative oddity at the end of World War II, it quickly became an important benefit for many workers (Starr 1982). By 1960, the United States was separating into two camps: the healthcare haves and have nots, as defined by access to insurance protection. The elderly contained a disproportionate share of the have nots.

Thus, covering senior citizens was a logical starting point for government action. The 1965 Medicare legislation represented one of the major hopes of President Lyndon Johnson's Great Society. However, Medicare had its origins in the proposals first put forward by President Harry Truman in the late 1940s, when he called for a national program to pay for medical care for all Americans (Marmor 1970). It is there we should go to understand how Medicare—in the form we know it today—came to be.

THE GENESIS

Medicare was signed into law on July 30, 1965, by President Johnson in a ceremony in Independence, Missouri, honoring the important role that President Harry Truman had played in the national health insurance debate in the years since World War II. Truman never saw passage of a national healthcare program during his presidency, but his advocacy set the ball rolling. Over time, the debate shifted to ensuring coverage for the elderly as the most vulnerable—and deserving—subgroup of the population. The election of President Johnson in 1964 set the stage for Medicare's passage.

Evolution of the Legislation

Public provision of health insurance was not popular during the administration of Dwight Eisenhower; employer-provided insurance continued to expand, and healthcare costs remained low. Nonetheless, the long history of support for public health insurance contains many Republican as well as Democratic supporters. For example, while governor of California, Republican Earl Warren proposed compulsory health insurance for the state in 1945 (Somers and Somers 1967). However, Republican opposition, coupled with the vociferous opposition of the American Medical Association (AMA), ended this and all other related national legislative initiatives through the 1950s.

The issue never died, however. A number of influential leaders in the field of social insurance, including Robert Ball, I. S. Falk, Wilbur Cohen, and union leader Nelson Cruikshank (from the American Federation of Labor), developed a bill that was introduced by Congressman Aime Forand of Rhode Island in 1957. Well-publicized hearings were held, and the bill, although failing to pass, represented the rallying point for the Democratic proposals in health (Campion 1984; Myers 1970). In 1959, President Eisenhower's secretary of Health, Education and Welfare, Arthur Flemming, released a report on options for providing hospital insurance to Social Security beneficiaries.

After supporting such legislation in the U.S. Senate, John F. Kennedy pledged in his presidential campaign to offer legislation for health insurance for the aged. Within a month of taking office, President Kennedy delivered to Congress a message calling for such legislation. Bills introduced by Congressman Cecil King of California and Senator Clinton Anderson of New Mexico became the focus of debate throughout the early 1960s (Marmor 1970).

But President Kennedy was unable to pass healthcare coverage for the elderly. Not until after his assassination did a more sympathetic environment for his proposals develop. The 1964 elections created a lopsided victory for the Democrats in Congress. In that period, President Johnson pushed Medicare and other Great Society legislation through Congress. With significant help from organized labor, which supported the legislation through its National Council of Senior Citizens, Medicare finally passed.

Even these efforts might not have prevailed without the "conversion" of Congressman Wilbur Mills. As the influential chairman of the House Ways and Means Committee, Mills was in a position to stop any legislation for health insurance. At first, Mills was not inclined to move; he had counted noses and did not have enough support in the House to pass the legislation. Mills was not a legislator who took on lost causes. But with President Johnson's landslide victory, some healthcare legislation seemed inevitable, so Mills took up the cause to control the outcome. Suspense then centered on what shape the plan would take.

Sensing that stonewalling was unlikely to work, opponents began to develop limited options. For example, the AMA, believing that the best it could achieve was to limit eligibility, lobbied relentlessly for restricting Medicare to the elderly poor. The AMA favored the Kerr-Mills Medical Assistance to the Aged approach (Derthick 1979), which would limit the size and influence of the public plan, effectively blocking it from becoming a mainstream healthcare program. The Republicans embraced this AMA alternative.

The supporters of Medicare viewed a means-tested approach as dangerous. One of the reasons for focusing first on the elderly had been to avoid creating a means-tested healthcare program.[3] Universal coverage offered the major political advantage of promising benefits for all, as had proven so popular with Social Security. Supporters felt this was crucial for Medicare as well.

The leaders stressed social insurance—that is, universal coverage paid for by broad-based taxes—and they went to considerable lengths to assert that all, or nearly all, the elderly had incomes too low to afford insurance (Marmor 1970). This was certainly an overstatement, but the claim was made to argue that it would not be worthwhile to means test the benefits.[4] Thus, the debate over means testing assumed a much broader significance, since both sides recognized that this issue would dramatically affect the public's perception of the plan and influence future policy moves in healthcare.

The breadth of services to be covered by this new health plan also became an issue. The King-Anderson bill, although making all the elderly eligible for benefits, was limited to hospital insurance. Proponents of social insurance saw the bill as a first step. Further benefits could be added later if the public accepted the concept of national insurance for hospital services for one portion of the population. However, supporters worried about the costs of the initial undertaking, so they proceeded cautiously.

Advocates of expanding coverage further came from both sides of the debate. Very liberal enthusiasts wanted fully comprehensive care. For example, the Forand bill, introduced in 1957, had been somewhat more inclusive, and other advocates went even further with their proposals. Ironically, the major proponents of broader coverage were the conservatives. The AMA/Republican strategy was to argue that it was better to comprehensively cover the poor than to only partially serve everyone. Consequently, their alternative bill was much more inclusive than the Democratic proposal in terms of covered services.

Together the two issues of eligibility and coverage could have stale-mated the entire process. For months the different parties wrangled and threatened to divide the interest groups lining up for and against various approaches. The AMA and the unions expended enormous sums to influence both public opinion and Congress. In retrospect, the elderly interest groups often cited as key players today lay low during these debates. Only the newly created National Council of Senior Citizens, which was effectively a subsidiary of the AFL-CIO, was prominent. The AARP, which already had a membership of more than 10 million in 1964, kept a conspicuously low profile. The AARP had testified in 1959 for a public-private partnership in which the Social Security system would serve only as a premium-collecting entity to help foster private insurance, such as its own Colonial Penn policies. It is notable that none of the major histories of Medicare tout significant roles for the AARP (Davis and Schoen 1978; Marmor 1970; Myers 1970; Skidmore 1970; Somers and Somers 1967). The players important in the later policy changes in Medicare thus are quite dif-ferent from those who led the first charge.

Medicare and Its Goals

The outcome stunned all observers. The final package put together by Mills went beyond what either side had proposed. Mills' solution to the impasse over the competing approaches was to establish two pro-grams: Medicare and Medicaid. Medicare would cover all those over 65 and would be divided into two parts: Part A, Hospital Insurance (plus skilled nursing care) and Part B, a voluntary, but subsidized, Supplementary Medical Insurance to cover primarily physician ser-vices. Medicaid would be targeted to low-income persons of all ages who were participating in other welfare programs.[5]

The basic structure of the Medicare program, with its large variety of benefits and patchwork of limitations and definitions, resulted from the negotiations between the House and the Senate. In particular, Senator Russell Long insisted on some changes to add further cata-strophic protections, and development of Part B drew from a proposal from Congressman John Byrnes (R-WI) (Myers 1970).[6] The outcome was a complicated structure of hospital benefits with coinsurance days and lifetime reserve days (defined in the appendix to this vol-ume). The legislation as finally passed in July 1965 had a starting date of July 1, 1966 (then the beginning of the federal fiscal year). From that date on, Medicare and Medicaid fundamentally transformed the shape of American healthcare. Rather than sinking Medicare, the opposition of the AMA not only helped create Medicaid but fostered an expanded scope of Medicare benefits (Marmor 1970).

The rules that were established to govern Medicare did little to disrupt or change the way healthcare was practiced or financed in the United States. Claims processing was structured to resemble that in the private sector. And Medicare statutes specifically assured free choice of provider and no interference in the routine practice of medicine. Payment rates were also designed to resemble those in the private sector, both in the mechanics and level of payment. Physicians' and other providers' groups that participated in the new program at least would not be put at a disadvantage. But even though the early emphasis was on ensuring that individuals would be covered and included in mainstream medical care, no one was sure that the AMA would not get the last laugh. Their ominous warnings about dangerous moves to socialized medicine carried the implicit threat that physicians might shun patients who were enrolled in either of these new programs. Indeed, in an article in the *New York Times* of August 12, 1965, the Association of American Physicians and Surgeons called for a boycott of Medicare.

But the new programs proved remarkably successful from the beginning. Large numbers of the elderly enrolled, and use of services expanded rapidly. There was no noticeable boycott by healthcare providers. By May 31, 1966, 17.6 million elderly persons had enrolled in the optional Part B plan—out of approximately 19 million who were eligible. And in the first three years of Medicare, about 100,000 eligible enrollees were admitted to hospitals each week (Myers 1970). Medicare led to a major increase in the elderly's use of medical care. Hospital discharges averaged 190 per 1,000 elderly persons in 1964 and 350 per 1,000 by 1973, for example, with most of the change occurring in the early years (Davis and Schoen 1978).[7] The proportion of the elderly using physician services jumped from 68 percent to 76 percent between 1963 and 1970 (Andersen et al. 1973).

Initially, everyone over the age of 65 was eligible. The legislation stressed access to care, without requiring a period of payroll tax contributions to achieve eligibility. This ensured a considerable windfall to persons aged 65 and older in 1966 and for many years thereafter. After the initial grandfathering of all the elderly, Medicare eligibility was limited to persons both over the age of 65 and entitled to Social Security benefits, either as workers or dependents. But the payroll contributions that persons in their late 50s and early 60s made into the Medicare trust fund in those early years did not nearly compensate for the costs of healthcare they received. Further, as costs of healthcare escalated into the 1970s, the costs of the program grew much faster than anticipated, and the "windfalls" to beneficiaries did not decline as anticipated.

For example, Health Care Financing Administration actuaries estimated that an elderly individual with average covered earnings retiring in 1982 would have paid in $2,200 and would have had $31,500 in expected future lifetime benefits—a ratio of 14.3 to 1 (Congressional Budget Office 1983). A more recent study has found that the contribution for an average worker retiring in 1991 would total $15,416, but that expected lifetime benefits would be $44,368—a ratio of 2.9 to 1 (Christensen 1992). Throughout the history of Medicare, payments into the system by workers have been far less than the ultimate returns in benefit payments, although the ratio of benefits to contributions is declining.[8]

EXPANSION IN 1972

The second major push for access to care extended Medicare coverage to disabled persons and to persons with end-stage renal disease (ESRD). Like coverage of the elderly, there was a considerable history of calls for expansion to disabled individuals. Coverage for this group had been recommended by the 1963–64 Advisory Council on Social Security. And although disabled persons were left out of the 1965 legislation, the Johnson administration proposed including them in 1967. Instead, a new advisory commission was set up that, in 1968, again recommended coverage. This commission advocated coverage of all disabled beneficiaries and insured workers who had been disabled for three months, resulting in a shorter waiting period than that for cash benefits (Myers 1970).

Ultimately, inclusion of disabled persons under Medicare came in 1972 as part of the sweeping Social Security amendments that substantially increased the commitments of all aspects of the program.[9] The disability expansion was added by Congress, however, and was not part of President Richard Nixon's proposed amendments (Derthick 1979).

One concession to holding down costs for disabled persons was to limit Medicare eligibility to disabled persons who had been receiving Social Security for at least two years. This meant that workers not only had to qualify as permanently and totally disabled (a condition for Social Security benefits, including a five-month waiting period), but they had to have stayed on the rolls for 24 months. Generally, eligibility for Social Security disability requires the worker to have paid payroll taxes for 20 out of the last 40 quarters (U.S. Social Security Administration 1991).[10]

The ESRD program was a last-minute addition to the Social Security amendments, but was not a new issue to Congress. Many bills had previously been offered to provide for treatment of end-stage renal disease, partly in response to the publicity war waged over the fact that this was a treatable disease for which treatment was largely unaffordable by average citizens (Rettig 1982). ESRD coverage was added by a floor amendment offered in the Senate at the end of the debate on the amendments, was then included in the conference report with less than 10 minutes of discussion, and hence became part of the final law (Rettig 1976).

Adding those with ESRD represented explicit coverage of a very visible group of persons with a specific, expensive ailment. Long-term kidney failure is fatal if the person does not receive dialysis (or a kidney transplant). Throughout the 1960s, growing attention was paid to the scarcity of kidney dialysis machines to treat patients. Waiting lists and rationing of this care highlighted a problem where patients were dying, not because there was no effective treatment but because of budget constraints and the resulting limited supply of dialysis machines.

The creation of a category of patients eligible for Medicare based solely on a particular condition caused many to worry that there might be a "disease of the month," so that gradually more and more people would be made eligible for coverage. Indeed, the numbers of kidney dialysis patients expanded far more rapidly than many expected. Although ESRD was a highly visible and expensive problem area, it was by no means unique as an expensive, deadly disease. But other groups have not been added in this way to Medicare, perhaps in part because of how expensive the ESRD patients have been over the last 20 years.[11] By 1993, the number of ESRD patients had grown to 237,000, at an average annual cost of over $30,000 per beneficiary (HCFA 1995).

The two groups thus added to Medicare's rolls resulted in an instant expansion of 10 percent in the number of beneficiaries and an even larger boost to the costs of the program, since disabled persons tend to be more expensive to cover than the elderly, on average (Ways and Means 1992). The impact of these new beneficiaries can clearly be seen in figure 2.1, which tracks the rate of growth in Medicare beneficiaries over time.

Figure 2.1 ANNUAL PERCENTAGE CHANGE IN NUMBER OF MEDICARE
ENROLLEES: CY1967–1993

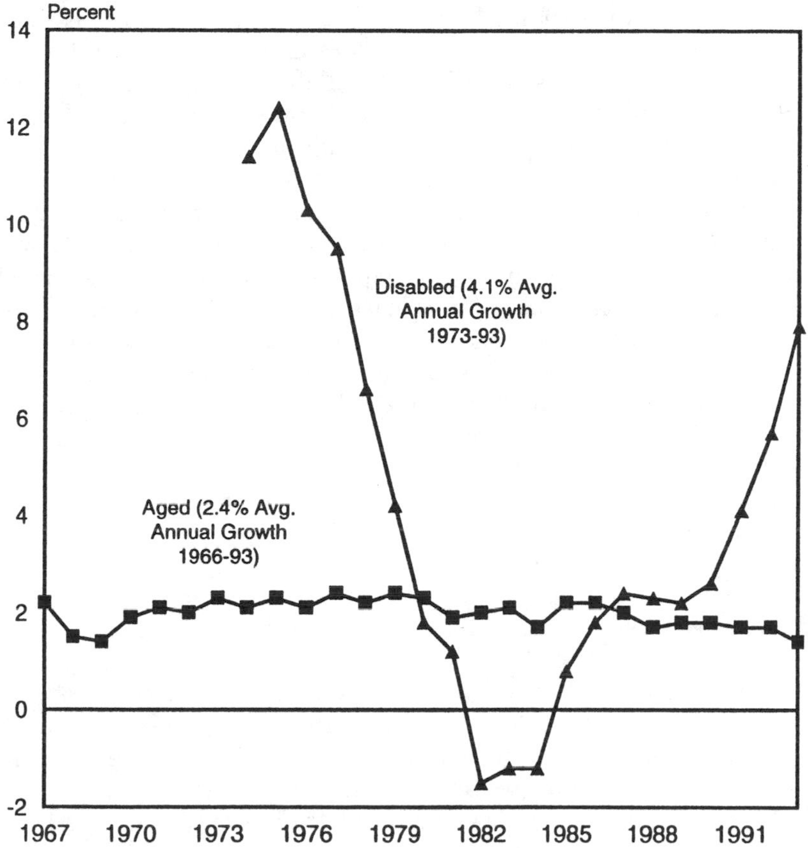

Source: HCFA (1995).

OTHER CHANGES IN ACCESS

Since 1972, Medicare has not been extended to any other broad group;
indeed, changes that affect coverage have largely represented fine-
tuning efforts at the margins, often to *restrict* access to the program.
At least thus far, Medicare has not served as the first step toward
national health insurance. Indeed, after serious debate in the 1970s,
the issue was largely set aside until the late 1980s.

Changes after 1972 reflect the shift away from access toward cost containment. Take the case of "expansion" of Medicare to all federal workers, which was passed as part of the Tax Equity and Fiscal Responsibility Act (TEFRA) of 1982 (Ways and Means 1985). Initially, Medicare coverage was not offered to federal workers, since they had their own healthcare system. In practice, however, many federal workers became eligible for Medicare through other means. In some cases their spouses were eligible and they became entitled by virtue of being elderly dependents of covered workers. Moreover, many federal workers have shifted between the private and the public sector over the course of their working lives. Consequently, they might have contributed very little but qualify for at least the minimum Social Security benefit and the full range of Medicare benefits. This "expansion" to new federal workers was thus actually a budget-reduction effort, requiring that all such workers pay the Medicare portion of the FICA tax for their full working lives. A similar expansion in 1986 included all newly hired state and local workers.

Other TEFRA legislation limited eligibility for the working elderly (aged 65 to 69), also as a budget-reducing measure. This legislation dictated that Medicare be the "secondary payer" for employed persons who have access to employer-provided health insurance. Private insurance was made responsible for paying most of an individual's healthcare bills, with Medicare paying only for those services not otherwise covered. The intent of this change was to reduce federal Medicare spending while not lowering insurance coverage for beneficiaries. These workers are guaranteed at least all the benefits offered by Medicare. The only question is who pays for that coverage.

During the 1980s the Reagan administration moved to *restrict* access by enforcing tougher eligibility standards for disability under Social Security. Any restriction on access to the cash-benefit program spills over to Medicare by also reducing the number of individuals who become eligible for Medicare. These efforts substantially slowed the rate of growth in the number of new disability beneficiaries during the 1980s (see figure 2.1). From 1975 to 1981, growth in disability beneficiaries averaged 5.6 percent per year. However, growth came to a virtual standstill between 1981 and 1986, after which eligibility grew slightly again. Over the entire 1981 to 1989 period, growth in the number of disability beneficiaries averaged just 0.7 percent annually (Ways and Means 1991). In the early 1990s disability enrollments again accelerated but have recently begun to moderate.

All of these changes were very limited, reflecting the retrenchment from expanding access at the beginning of the program. No major cuts have occurred in the two major groups covered by Medicare, although proposals in this area are now receiving more discussion.

The one important exception to these trends was the Qualified Medicare Beneficiary (QMB) program, which was instituted as part of the Medicare catastrophic legislation and survived its repeal. This program covers Medicare cost sharing and Part B premiums for anyone with an income below the poverty level ($7,740 for an individual in 1996). A related program also covers those between 100 percent and 120 percent of poverty, but only for the cost of the Part B premium. Thus far, however, participation rates have been low, since individuals must apply through the Medicaid program for the benefits, and states have not been anxious to publicize it (Families USA 1992). But recent analysis of the numbers of Medicare beneficiaries with any type of Medicaid coverage indicates a 4.3 percentage point rise between 1987 and 1991 (Chulis et al. 1993). And between 1993 and 1996, HCFA reports the number of QMB enrollees specifically rose from 4.2 million to 4.8 million.

WHO GETS WHAT?

Although the eligibility and scope of Medicare have remained basically the same and reflect uniform national benefits, the impact of Medicare still varies widely across individuals. In particular, the relatively high cost-sharing requirements of Medicare constrain the ability of vulnerable groups to utilize Medicare coverage. Karen Davis (1975) has long argued forcefully for improved protections from cost sharing, and has pointed out access problems for minority groups, for the low-income elderly, and for persons residing in certain regions of the country. If such persons do not use services, even though they are entitled to them, because of prohibitive out-of-pocket costs or supply problems, then Medicare is less universal than it appears on paper.

Thus, a discussion of access issues flows naturally into a concern about who gets what from Medicare. Such analysis could focus on a wide range of demographic indicators. For example, women tend to use more chronic care services, compared to men's heavier use of acute care. Since Medicare has done a poorer job of covering these chronic care services, women's coverage under Medicare in any given year is less generous than that for men—a difference that has persisted over time. On the other hand, Sandra Christensen (1992) has also pointed out that women's longer life expectancy raises their lifetime expected benefits enough to overshadow these annual differences. Participation by minorities is also a concern in Medicare, although the numbers of persons served show smaller differences by racial category today than in the early years of the program (HCFA 1995).

This discussion focuses on the two most important indicators of who gets what from Medicare: income and location.

Rising Burdens of Medicare Cost Sharing

Medicare cost sharing formally includes deductibles assessed under both Parts A and B of the program and coinsurance for many of the services provided. Coinsurance requires beneficiaries to pay a percentage of the costs of the service. The largest source of cost sharing is usually from the coinsurance on physician services. Extra billing by physicians for charges above what Medicare designates as reasonable also constitutes a form of cost sharing. Finally, Part B premiums, although technically not cost sharing, constitute a substantial payment burden for those with moderate incomes. Table 2.1 contains an average per capita breakdown for these components.

The impact of increases in Medicare cost sharing over time has fallen disproportionately on those with low incomes who lack access to the Medicaid program. The RAND Corporation health insurance experiment of the 1970s indicated that cost sharing serves as a deterrent to use of services for persons with low or moderate incomes (Newhouse et al. 1982). Although that study contained no elderly persons, the striking results of a differential impact by family income would certainly carry over to Medicare beneficiaries. A $20 coinsur-

Table 2.1 COMPONENTS OF MEDICARE COST SHARING, 1993

	Average per Capita ($)
Part A	211
Deductibles	148
Coinsurance	62
Part B	858
Deductibles	81
Coinsurance	324
Balance Billing	14
Premiums	439
Total	1,069

Sources: Data extrapolated from Health Care Financing Administration, 1995.

ance payment for a physician visit is simply more burdensome to someone whose income is $8,000 a year than to someone with $20,000 or $40,000 a year.

Many researchers have observed variations in the use of services by the elderly of varying income levels. For example, Christensen and Kasten (1988a) noted that Medicare benefits per enrollee generally rise with income, from $2,052 for the bottom 10 percent of the income distribution to a high of over $2,800 for those in the top half of the distribution. These differences persist even after controlling for health status (Feder et al. 1987a).

Relief is available for persons eligible for Medicaid. Medicaid fills in where Medicare leaves off, paying the required cost sharing and adding other benefits. But less than half of the elderly poor receive Medicaid. States restrict eligibility to hold down costs by keeping income and assets limits very restrictive. Even the QMB program only partly solves the problems of high cost sharing. This program includes those with incomes below 100 percent of poverty. For anyone above the poverty level up to 120 percent, help is limited to covering the Part B premium through the companion Specified Low Income Beneficiary Program. Individuals still have to pay for other cost sharing out of pocket.

The affordability issue extends well beyond the poverty level. Medicare enrollees averaged $1,069 in out-of-pocket liabilities just for Medicare-covered services in 1993 (HCFA 1995). Someone with an income of even 150 percent of the poverty level would have to contribute over 9 percent of his or her income to pay just for the average amount of required cost sharing under Medicare. And that individual would likely owe at least another 12 percent or more for noncovered services (Moon and Mulvey 1995). This person would be ineligible for help from Medicaid or the QMB program.

This calculation becomes bleaker each year as the costs of medical care—and hence the burdens on beneficiaries—rise. For example, as figure 2.2 shows, Medicare cost sharing is consuming an ever-increasing portion of the income of the elderly—and the story is likely to be the same for disabled persons as well. Thus, problems of access attributable to the burdens of cost sharing will almost surely continue for those of moderate means.

In practice, many of the elderly buy or receive as part of retirement benefits supplemental insurance to help pay for this cost sharing. Those who receive employer-subsidized coverage are at least partially protected from out-of-pocket costs; they have their cost sharing cov-

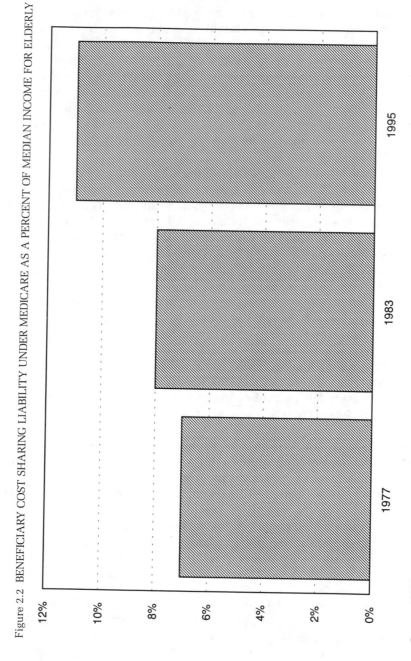

Figure 2.2 BENEFICIARY COST SHARING LIABILITY UNDER MEDICARE AS A PERCENT OF MEDIAN INCOME FOR ELDERLY

Source: HCFA (1995a); U.S. Bureau of the Census (1996).

ered and do not have to pay the full premium costs for the protection. In 1991, this group constituted about 38 percent of all the elderly (Chulis et al. 1993).

But purchasing "Medigap" insurance is not a solution for high average healthcare burdens. Such insurance can reduce the annual variation in the burden for moderate-income Medicare beneficiaries, but it actually raises average costs. Medigap adds to the costs of care, since purchasers of this supplemental insurance pay for the marketing and administrative costs and (in some cases) profits for insurers, in addition to the average costs of healthcare. In practice, this amounts to at least 20 percent to 30 percent above the expected benefits in premiums and sometimes much more (Shikles 1990). If the problem of high cost sharing were confined to a few high-cost patients, supplemental insurance would help. However, Medigap cannot solve the problem, since even the median costs of Medicare-related liabilities are unaffordable for most moderate-income enrollees.

Geographic Variation

Variation in the supply of providers across areas of the United States also restricts access of enrollees to Medicare benefits. Access problems may reflect where enrollees live, such as isolated rural areas where the population is too small to support certain services. Or, these problems may be related to enrollee incomes. If the enrollee lives in a poor area, providers may not be located nearby. In some areas where costs have risen rapidly and Medicare payments have not kept pace, providers may be reluctant to see Medicare patients. These geographic factors result in eligible persons who need Medicare services not getting access to care.

The large variations observed around the United States in receipt of Medicare services at least in part reflect these supply problems. In other cases, such variations in use of services reflect different medical practices that may or may not be indicators of major problems for patients. In 1993, for example, state-by-state breakdowns of the number of enrollees served by Medicare ranged from a low of 604 per 1,000 enrollees in Hawaii to a high of 904 per 1,000 in Iowa. Reimbursement per person served ranged from $3,029 in Nebraska to $6,607 in the District of Columbia (HCFA 1995). If enrollees are divided into urban versus rural areas, Part B allowed charges indicate that urban enrollees had 31 percent higher expenditures than their rural counterparts in 1988 (Holahan unpublished data). Although some of the difference in dollars of expenditures reflects different payment levels around the country, use of services also differs substantially.

Medicare calculates the average per capita costs for its beneficiaries for each county in the United States. Table 2.2 shows these amounts for elderly beneficiaries in the five highest and five lowest cost counties for 1996. While costs generally are highest in urban areas such as New York City, and lowest in very rural areas, that is not always the case. In fact, in 1996, the highest per capita cost is for Loving, Texas—a sparsely populated rural county in the panhandle.[12] What is most striking in this table is the very wide differences across counties, reflecting differences of more than four to one from highest to lowest. Such great differences create important challenges for a universal program like Medicare.

CONCLUSIONS

By most accounts, Medicare has improved access to healthcare by the nation's elderly and disabled populations. By 1970, it had enrolled nearly all of the elderly and, by 1974, a substantial number of America's disabled in a national healthcare program. Providing these pop-

TABLE 2.2 AVERAGE ANNUAL PER CAPITA COST OF MEDICARE FOR PERSONS AGED 65+ FOR SELECTED COUNTIES, 1996

County	Monthly amount		
	Part A	Part B	Total
Highest Five			
Loving, TX	$698	$183	$881
Richmond, NY	$538	$221	$759
Bronx, NY	$529	$204	$734
New York, NY	$490	$225	$715
Kings, NY	$486	$217	$703
Lowest Five			
Fall River, SD	$132	$75	$207
Banner, NE	$104	$107	$211
Saline, NE	$131	$86	$217
Holmes, OH	$134	$83	$217
Presidio, TX	$135	$84	$219
National Median	$235	$126	$364
National Average	$238	$129	$372

Source: HCFA (1996a).

ulation groups with access to mainstream medical care resulted in a dramatic rise in service use.

But the goal of ensuring access to mainstream care has not yet been fully achieved. The other side of the story is that although Medicare offers universal coverage under a uniform federal program, use of services varies dramatically across beneficiaries. Access remains a problem for those with low incomes, for whom the costs of out-of-pocket expenses remain a substantial barrier to access. This is attested to by variations in use that extend beyond what would be expected by differences in health status. A different set of problems besets those who reside in certain underserved areas—both rural and urban settings. Again, use varies substantially—beyond what one might expect as a reasonable difference in attitudes toward care or need for services.

But access problems for particular groups aside, Medicare finances a great deal of health care. In 1996, the average Medicare beneficiary will receive about $4,300 in services under the program. Medicare's very "success" contributed to the rapid growth in federal costs to maintain it. Thus was ushered in the second "phase" of Medicare—a concern for cost containment—which is the subject of the next two chapters.

Notes

1. In 1950 the Old Age Assistance program had also established a system of vendor payments to providers of healthcare for the elderly, but with even more limited federal dollars.

2. Some states continued their MAA programs after 1965, as allowed by law in lieu of Medicaid for the elderly. MAA was eliminated in 1969.

3. Ironically, accounts of this debate indicating concerns that means testing would undermine public support for Medicare sound very similar to the more recent controversy over the Medicare Catastrophic Coverage Act (see chapter 5).

4. However, health coverage was not, in turn, a major focus of those concerned about poverty per se during this period. To these groups, healthcare needs were an important, but not an extraordinary, concern. They emphasized income adequacy as the key to affordability of all basic goods and services. Healthcare's cost spiral had not yet become so great a concern.

5. Medicaid is, like MAA, a joint federal/state program in which the federal government sets some rules and provides matching monies to states. The states must provide benefits to those eligible for cash assistance. Certain benefits are federally mandated. Beyond that, the states may choose to cover additional services and additional beneficiaries under the medically needy provision. Medicaid is available to persons of all ages. Over time, its importance for the elderly has been primarily for long-term care services not

covered by Medicare and as a supplemental program filling Medicare's gaps for those with very low incomes.

6. Senator Long also argued for means-tested cost sharing. Although that provision was not included in the legislation, it is interesting that the issues raised by Long began to resurface in the late 1980s as a potential direction for change in Medicare.

7. Indeed, the system was so successful that critics both then and later pointed to the danger of increasing costs of healthcare—a criticism that proved well founded. Perhaps the AMA got the last laugh after all. A *New York Times* article of August 19, 1966, indicated that physicians' prices for the elderly rose by 300 percent on the introduction of Medicare.

8. This ratio is likely to decline even faster now for those who pay at the maximum, since the cap on earnings subject to the tax increased in 1991.

9. The 1972 amendments also allowed individuals over the age of 65 to buy in to Part A if they were not otherwise eligible, and established a few minor expansions of services. These amendments also raised the Part B deductible from $50 to $60 and, in what would become an important change over time, tied premium increases in Part B to the newly added Social Security cost of living adjustment (COLA) (U.S. Social Security Administration 1991).

10. Younger workers have lesser requirements, and persons in other categories such as disabled adult children must meet other standards.

11. This issue has again been raised in the context of eligibility for the AIDS population. Many AIDS victims will die before becoming eligible for Medicare through the traditional disability program. Advocates for AIDS patients thus urge that, as is now the case for ESRD, there should be no waiting period.

12. It is likely that this reflects the influence of a small number of very high-cost cases.

Chapter Three

CONTAINING COSTS:
IMPACTS ON PROVIDERS

It was not long before Medicare began to be viewed with alarm, not because of its failure, but because of its success. The rapid initial growth in the cost of the program testifies to how quickly the system began to fulfill its original goal of offering mainstream medical care to older persons. The addition of disabled and end-stage renal disease patients in 1972 further enlarged program costs.

It is not surprising, then, that the second major "phase" of Medicare focused almost exclusively on controlling program costs. Indeed, immediately after passage, many observers were already expressing concern at Medicare's growth. Healthcare costs received attention from President Richard Nixon during the period of wage and price controls. Predictions of Medicare's "bankruptcy" also began to surface. In 1970, Chief Actuary Robert Myers predicted an enormous deficit in Medicare for 1995 (Feder 1977). The 1981 report on the Federal Hospital Insurance Trust Fund indicated that the fund would be in deficit by 1991 (HI Trustees 1981). These projections of future spending indicated that something had to give, that higher taxes or lower spending would be necessary to keep the Medicare trust fund solvent.

Worry over costs in the 1970s spurred a number of cost-containment efforts. However, it was the prospect of enormous federal deficits and efforts to reduce them that provided the executive and legislative branches with additional impetus for major cost-containment measures in the decade following. By 1980, Medicare was the second largest federal domestic program and the fastest growing one, making it a target for those concerned about the size of government in general. Decisions about Medicare in the 1980s thus reflected general concern not only about rising healthcare costs but also about the size of the federal budget deficit.

Under each budget submission by the Reagan administration, Medicare cost cutting was accorded a central place in proposals to reduce the size of the federal budget deficit. Policy was as much budget-driven as centered on devising innovative new approaches to provider payments. Nonetheless, many of the cost-containment strategies chosen have revolutionized the way we pay providers in the United States, and Medicare often has been used as a model for other payers seeking to hold down costs.

Enthusiasm for cost cutting within Medicare extended to all aspects of the program. Most of the emphasis centered on reducing payments to providers of Medicare services, but beneficiaries also faced reductions in benefits and increased requirements for cost sharing. A study by the Congressional Budget Office (1991) concluded that in 1990, Medicare spending was 20 percent below what it would have been without the changes of the 1980s. Nonetheless, throughout the 1980s, Medicare maintained its distinction as the fastest growing domestic federal program. And although there have been fewer changes passed in the 1990s to reduce Medicare spending, that goal continues to rank high on the agenda of many policymakers.

This chapter examines these increasing costs and assesses major cost-containment efforts that have been directed at the provider level, especially with regard to hospitals and physician services. Chapter 4 addresses the impacts of cost-containment efforts on beneficiaries.

SOURCES OF GROWTH IN MEDICARE SPENDING

Expenditures on all parts of Medicare have risen dramatically. Like the growth in aggregate healthcare spending, Medicare expenditures reflect both price inflation and increases in the use of services. Hospital expenditures led the way in the 1970s, and physician spending took off in the 1980s. Although use of services contributed to this growth, the bottom line is that prices were responsible for considerable growth in the late 1970s, making price controls a natural place to start any cost-containment strategy.

Table 3.1 provides breakdowns for the major components of expenditure growth for the two parts of Medicare over four periods: 1967–74, 1974–83, 1983–90, and 1990–93. The first period coincided with the highest growth in the number of enrollees in the program. Reimbursements grew rapidly as well, particularly for hospital care, a trend that intensified in the 1974 to 1983 period. From 1974 to 1983, per enrollee expenditures, which are the combination of persons served and reimbursement per person served, grew more than 15 percent per year, on average (HCFA 1995). It was not until the post-1983 period

Table 3.1 AVERAGE ANNUAL PERCENTAGE CHANGES IN MEDICARE, 1967–93

	Hospital Insurance			Supplementary Medical Insurance		
Period	Growth in Number of Enrollees	Growth in Persons Served per 1,000 Enrollees	Growth in Reimburse-ments per Person Served	Growth in Number of Enrollees	Growth in Persons Served per 1,000 Enrollees	Growth in Reimburse-ments per Person Served
1967–74	3.0%	0.8%	11.0%	3.8%	4.4%	5.1%
1974–83	2.4	1.8	13.5	2.5	3.5	13.7
1983–90	1.9	−2.6	8.9	1.7	3.0	7.4
1990–93	2.1	0.8	6.4	2.0	0.8	3.6

Source: HCFA (1995).

that growth rates slowed down, even though there was considerable cost-containment legislation passed from 1981 through 1983. After 1983, growth slowed in both the proportion of beneficiaries using services and in their average expenditures. It should also be noted that this was a period of decline in overall inflation rates compared to the late 1970s and early 1980s.

The figures in table 3.1 also help to identify the sources of the rapidly rising Medicare costs. Growth in numbers of enrollees has been a declining factor since 1974. For Part A, consisting mainly of hospital services, growth in the proportion of enrollees using services was also a limited contributor to the problem. Indeed after 1984, the rate of enrollees using services fell substantially, particularly for hospital and skilled nursing facility (SNF) care.[1] It picked up again after 1990, but is rising only slowly. But Part A reimbursements per beneficiary using services grew rapidly—at a rate of nearly 14 percent from 1974 to 1983. These changes reflect both rising prices and increasing intensity of services offered in the hospital. Each year, more tests and services were performed, but more important, the prices were higher.

Figure 3.1 illustrates the impact of inflation, showing the growth of Hospital Insurance (HI) costs per enrollee in nominal dollars and after adjusting for inflation, using two alternative indices. The overall consumer price index (CPI) offers an adjustment that indicates what happened to Part A spending relative to constant purchasing power. That adjustment indicates that the general rate of inflation, which was extremely high in the late 1970s and early 1980s, accounted for a substantial share of the higher Part A spending per enrollee.

If the spending figure is adjusted, instead, for the rate of price increases just in healthcare goods and services, the growth line is flatter still. This means that much of the growth in per capita spend-

Figure 3.1 PER ENROLLEE HI BENEFIT PAYMENTS ADJUSTED BY ALTERNATIVE PRICE DEFLATORS, 1975–95

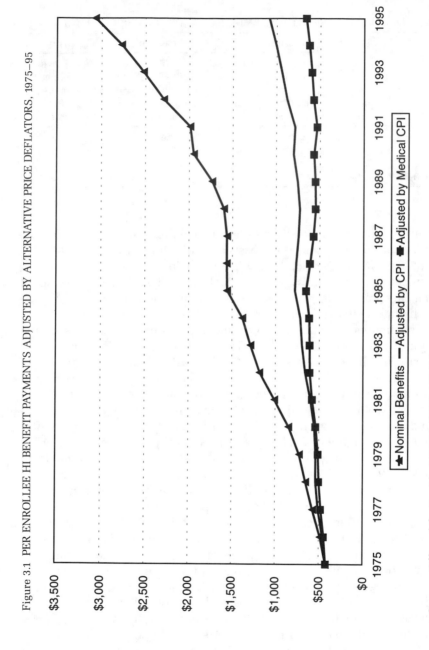

Sources: Office of the President (1996); HCFA (1996b).

ing on Medicare Part A can be attributed to healthcare inflation. This comparison is most relevant for the 1975–82 period, before Medicare prices began to be controlled. After that point, Medicare was permitted lower rates of growth in payments than occurred in the economy as a whole.[2]

Thus, not unexpectedly, much of the emphasis in cost control for hospital care centered on controlling the price of care. The blank-check approach of the original legislation was always of concern to those who worried about program costs. Hospitals were essentially paid on the basis of what they spent on Medicare beneficiaries. Long lengths of stay and redundant services were rewarded with higher levels of reimbursement to hospitals.

The picture is somewhat different for Part B (Supplementary Medical Insurance [SMI]); costs continued to grow, overtaking the rate of growth in Part A after 1984. This part of the program shows much more substantial growth in the number of persons receiving benefits each year. The low level of the SMI deductible, raised only twice between 1973 and 1993, meant that price inflation increased substantially the number of enrollees exceeding the deductible limit and hence receiving benefits each year. By 1993, almost 81 percent of all Medicare enrollees exceeded the deductible amount, compared to 52 percent in 1975 (HCFA 1995). Reimbursements per person grew at a slower rate after 1983, but were above 7 percent annually through 1990 (table 3.1). After 1990, these rates also slowed substantially, capturing the early effects of physician payment reform.

Prices also played a major role in SMI growth, as indicated in figure 3.2. Again three growth lines are shown: the top line uses dollars uncorrected for inflation, the middle line corrects for general inflation in the economy, and the bottom indicates growth after accounting for price increases in physician services. Again, the bottom line is most relevant before Medicare policy began to restrict price growth. Before 1984, price growth in Medicare largely mirrored that for physician services as a whole.

Since 1984, Congress has set the maximum annual rate of increase in physician payments by law and has used that as a policy lever to control costs of Part B services. The mechanism was the Medicare Economic Index (MEI), which sets limits on the rate of growth of Medicare's prevailing charges for physicians.[3] For example, beginning on July 1, 1984, the MEI was frozen for 16 months. Thus the MEI in the last half of the 1980s was considerably lower than the overall rate of inflation for such services. Nonetheless, this line in figure 3.2 is not as flat as that for the hospital side of Medicare, shown in figure

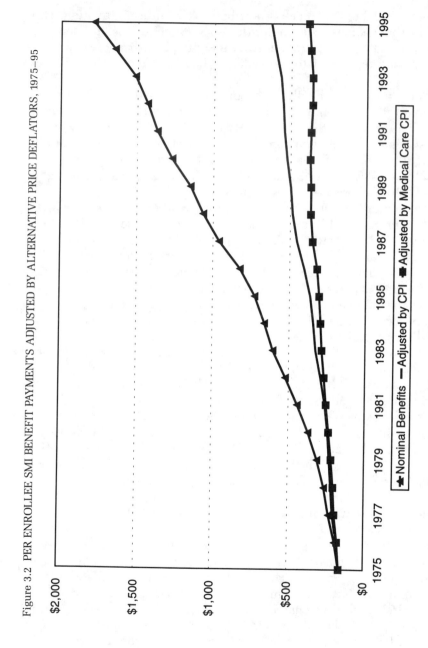

Figure 3.2 PER ENROLLEE SMI BENEFIT PAYMENTS ADJUSTED BY ALTERNATIVE PRICE DEFLATORS, 1975–95

★ Nominal Benefits — Adjusted by CPI ■ Adjusted by Medical Care CPI

Sources: Office of the President (1996); HCFA (1996b).

3.1, indicating more real growth in the use and intensity of services in the physician services part of Medicare.

CHANGING MEDICARE'S RELATIONSHIP WITH PROVIDERS

When Medicare was enacted in 1965, much of the debate on implementation centered on achieving the confidence of hospitals and physicians. Mainstream medical care would be offered to older persons only if the program could overcome the stigma of "socialized medicine" and the rancorous debate over passage. Because of these concerns, Medicare was set up to operate as much like private insurance as possible. Private insurance companies were selected to process the claims (referred to as "carriers" for Part B and "intermediaries" for Part A). Generally, a different company served each state, ensuring that physicians and hospitals would deal with familiar faces. The rules for processing claims were decentralized, creating considerable area variation. Carriers and intermediaries enjoyed (and still have) great latitude in their relationships with healthcare providers concerning claims processing.

In the early years of Medicare, physicians, in particular, were subject to almost no controls on the care they provided, nor on billing practices. This was done in large part to reassure physicians and to guarantee their acceptance of Medicare. Doctors used whatever forms they had used before Medicare's passage. At their option, they could either bill Medicare directly for each service or bill the patient. Although Medicare established limits on what the government would pay (called allowed charges), physicians were free to bill the patient the full amount of their actual charge, collecting any difference between actual and allowed charges from the patient. Moreover, because Medicare's allowed charges were computed in much the same way that Blue Cross/Blue Shield calculated reasonable charges, they were not much of a restraining force.

Over time, Medicare's allowed charges strongly reflected the historical rates in various areas—rates that were not very responsive to changes in the general market for physicians' services or to changes in technology that made procedures simpler or more complex over time. A number of interim steps were taken to modify the payment structure. But until physician payment reform passed in late 1989, Medicare physician payment schedules were largely based on historical patterns established in 1966.

Hospitals were also treated generously in the beginning of the Medicare program. They were allowed to bill on a cost basis with no oversight about the appropriateness of the services rendered. But hospitals were the first to be subjected to stringent cost controls—in part because of the rapid growth in costs in this sector, but also because the sector is the largest and most formally organized part of the health-care system. Policymakers felt they had a handle on hospitals' behavior and could thus seek to mold it over time.

HOSPITALS TAKE THE FIRST HIT

From 1965 to 1974, Medicare paid hospitals on the principle of "reasonable and necessary costs." Hospitals had to fill out detailed cost reports and face auditing of their expenses, but essentially they billed Medicare for whatever services were provided. These were not the published charges that hospitals generally apply to patients, but were costs for each hospital as calculated by Medicare's intermediaries. Hospitals could not charge whatever they liked, but once costs were established, there were no constraints on the amount of care provided.

Although this was the initial bargain struck to help secure Medicare's passage, debate began almost immediately on how to control hospital costs. But although the concern was there, consensus on major reform was lacking (Feder 1977). Robert Myers (1970) noted, however, that even in the first several years of Medicare there was interest in a per capita payment system for hospitals.

A number of more limited constraints were introduced over this period. In 1972, Professional Standards Review Organizations (PSROs) were established to review and control beneficiaries' use of services (Feder et al. 1982). Beginning in 1974, a reimbursement cap was added to prevent any hospital from charging more than 120 percent of the mean of routine costs found in similar facilities. Thus, this first constraint on hospitals required them to hold their costs in line with those of other hospitals in the area. Over time, this limit (called a "223" limit after its Social Security statute) was ratcheted downward to 112 percent (Office of Technology Assessment 1985). But this approach did not force major efficiencies on hospitals, since they were still being paid on the basis of what they spent, and the limits applied only to basic services.

In 1974 and 1975, Hospital Insurance payments grew at rates in excess of 20 percent, prompting the administration of Jimmy Carter to propose national hospital rate setting (Feder et al. 1982). This dramatic proposal was defeated when hospitals pledged voluntarily to hold down costs. During consideration of that legislation, hospital cost growth did slow substantially, even though the period was generally marked by very high rates of overall inflation. But the impact proved only temporary. In 1980 and 1981, growth rates in HI once more approached 20 percent, even though inflation was abating elsewhere (see figure 3.3). No longer could the industry credibly argue that it could police itself.

The confluence of efforts to cut Medicare spending as part of general budget reductions and concerns about rampant growth in the hospital sector made hospitals an obvious target for budget cuts in the 1980s. Since over two-thirds of Medicare payments went to hospitals, they were the place "where the money was." Medicare cost cutting for hospitals in the 1980s did not start with the Prospective Payment System (PPS), as many believe; its origins were earlier. The Omnibus Budget Reconciliation Act of 1981 tightened the "223" limits on what hospitals could receive as reimbursement for routine operating costs to 108 percent of mean costs (Office of Technology Assessment 1985). That is, a hospital could receive no more than 108 percent of costs averaged across all similar hospitals. But this was only the beginning.

Substantially more stringent restrictions were added by the Tax Equity and Fiscal Responsibility Act of 1982 (TEFRA). TEFRA expanded the 223 limits, and added a new hospital-specific target rate on costs per case.[4] The initial 120 percent limit was scheduled to be reduced over three years to 110 percent. But the most important change was that these limits would no longer be based on spending each year, but rather on costs up to a ceiling trended forward through time. This meant that each year the restrictions would be more severe and more binding (Office of Technology Assessment 1985). Impacts on spending growth were considerable (figure 3.3).

TEFRA also introduced several new concepts into hospital reimbursement. First, the per case limits moved away from retrospective payments to a payment schedule set in advance. TEFRA replaced the old per diem approach to hospital payment with a per case approach and permitted hospitals to benefit, at least partially, from any cost savings they generated.[5] For the first time, hospitals had incentives to seek efficiencies in the provision of care.

But the stringent TEFRA limits left hospitals without enough flexibility to benefit from the efficiencies they introduced. The climate set by the TEFRA limits led many hospitals to conclude that almost any other plan would be preferable, thereby smoothing the way for

Figure 3.3 ANNUAL RATES OF GROWTH IN MEDICARE HOSPITAL PAYMENTS, 1975–93

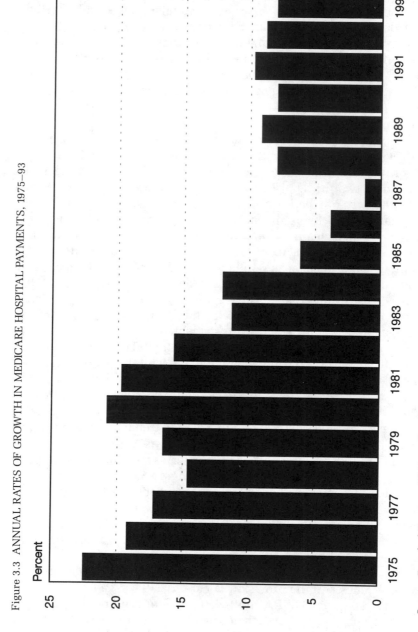

Source: Board of Trustees, HI Trust Fund (1990, 1993, and 1995).

introduction of radical payment reform. Indeed, TEFRA itself called for the U.S. Department of Health and Human Services (DHHS) to devise a new plan for reimbursing hospitals, indicating that TEFRA changes were meant as interim rules.

This new hospital payment reform was implemented quickly. The DHHS presented its proposal to Congress in December 1982, with many unresolved details left open for negotiation. Some pundits predicted that prolonged debate and lobbying would delay passage. The Reagan administration and Congress worked feverishly in the spring of 1983 to hash out the compromise that led to the legislation. Although the DHHS and the Congressional Budget Office put considerable effort into analyzing the impacts on hospitals of various alternatives, the deadlines for enactment dictated that many of the adjustments were ad hoc and many of the potential specific impacts remained unclear.

The new legislation, called the Prospective Payment System (PPS), came into being in April 1983. Because PPS was tied to critical legislation to protect the solvency of the Social Security system, the PPS amendments received less attention than if they had been proposed as standalone legislation. The final details were not debated or subjected to the scrutiny of interest groups, which might have slowed the process.

PPS began as a great experiment in systemwide reform, with no one certain of the outcome. In fact, Congress also established a Prospective Payment Assessment Commission (ProPAC) to oversee the implementation of this complicated new system and advise on the inevitable changes that would be necessary to fine-tune it over time. PPS counts as a major coup for Congress and the administration, even given the continuing concerns described in the next section. It radically changed payment policy to hospitals with a minimum of disruption to the healthcare system.

How PPS Works

The basic justification for PPS was a desire to stop paying hospitals on the basis of costs already incurred. Such a system was widely recognized as contributing to health inflation, since hospitals had no incentive to seek more efficient ways to provide care. To reward efficiency, PPS needed not only to move away from a cost-plus system but to establish a payment mechanism that was not only sensitive to legitimate differences in costs of care but also one that hospitals could understand. The presumption was that a system was needed that would pay a fixed amount set in advance for services (Russell 1989). Further, such a system would be based on national or regional rates and not the costs of the individual hospitals. Hospitals with lower than average costs would be rewarded, whereas those with higher costs would be forced to economize. The payment levels also needed to reflect differences in patients, in types of services offered, and in variations in input prices over which hospitals had no control. Since hospital services vary dramatically—from simple procedures performed on relatively healthy individuals to highly complex treatments or surgery on individuals with multiple, complicated health problems—the system had to be flexible enough to change over time as medical practice and patient needs also changed. And it must not encourage hospitals to respond merely by admitting only lower-cost patients.

PPS established payment schedules for hospitals by setting prices per diagnosis. Patients are classified into a diagnosis-related group (DRG), and total payments to a hospital reflect the mix of patients as indicated by the DRGs.[6] In addition to separating patients into groups depending upon the problem for which they are admitted and the procedures performed, some attempt is made to identify patients requiring heavier care.[7] There is also special provision for additional payments to cover extraordinarily expensive cases.[8]

The DRG is assigned a weight indicating the level of hospital costs for persons in that group relative to a standard case. The weights, which help establish the prospective payment for the patient, are set nationally and reflect the costs of care for Medicare patients. For example, the weight for a simple appendectomy without complications was .7892 in 1996, compared to 16.3066 for a liver transplant or .4976 for an allergic reaction by a patient over the age of 17 (HCFA 1996c). Table 3.2 includes additional examples of the most common DRG groups and their weights.[9]

The actual payment level for a hospital reflects a multistep process, in which DRGs are only one component. First, the hospital is assigned a basic fee for a standardized case, calculated on the basis of the average cost of a hospital stay for that type of hospital (i.e., whether it is located in an urban, large urban, or rural area). The basic rate is then adjusted by the weight for the particular DRG into which the patient is classified. Adjustments to that rate are then also made—for example, for differences in local wages or for cases in which the hospital serves a disproportionate share of low-income patients, is the sole community hospital, or is a teaching hospital. Thus, whereas the

Table 3.2 MOST COMMON DRGs AND THEIR WEIGHTS

DRG[a] Number and Description	1993 Discharges (in thousands)	1996 Weight
Total DRGs	11,157.9	
127 Heart failure and shock	693.6	1.0302
089 Simple pneumonia and pleurisy[b]	431.2	1.1211
014 Specific cerebrovascular disorders except transient ischemic attack	354.2	1.2065
088 Chronic obstructive pulmonary disease	346.9	1.0018
140 Angina pectoris	315.4	0.6312
209 Major joint and limb reattachment procedures	309.2	2.2707
182 Esophagitis, gastroenteritis, and miscellaneous digestive disorders[b]	237.7	0.7794
430 Psychoses	237.6	0.8670
296 Nutritional and miscellaneous metabolic disorders[b]	230.5	0.9166
174 Gastrointestinal hemorrhage with cardiovascular complications	230.0	0.9880
138 Cardiac arrhythmia and conduction disorders with cardiovascular complications	203.1	0.8049
079 Respiratory infections and inflammations[b]	185.0	1.6625

Source: HCFA (1996c, 1995); HCFA (1995).
a. DRG, diagnosis-related group.
b. Age greater than 17, with complications.

rates are set nationally, considerable variation occurs as a result of the location or other characteristics of the hospital.[10]

The goal of PPS is to encourage hospitals to find efficient ways to deliver care. The payment calculated for a hospital for a particular DRG is made regardless of the actual costs of treating the patient. If hospitals are able to deliver care at less than the amount of the prospective payment, they may keep the difference. Furthermore, although hospitals may lose on particular patients or in particular DRG categories, on average the hospital should be able to cover its costs—or even make a profit. The system was never designed to fully cover the costs of all patients in each DRG; rather, the gains and losses for individual cases are expected to even out over the year. Implicitly, the system also assumes that there are a sufficient number of cases within a hospital for the averaging to occur.

No longer is there an incentive to keep patients for long periods or to perform many procedures that will be reimbursed at cost. Rather, hospitals find it in their financial interest to limit lengths of stay and tests or procedures performed. The downside of such a system is the possibility that patients will be discharged too early (the "quicker and sicker" issue) and that necessary tests will not be performed. Thus, some of the simplest responses hospitals can make may put patients at risk. Further, hospitals may find it beneficial to discourage admission of high-cost patients within particular DRGs or patients with certain DRGs that are costly to that hospital.[11]

The other major problem anticipated by the legislation was the likelihood of "DRG creep." This could arise if hospitals were to "game" the system by assigning patients to DRGs with the highest possible weights. But such gaming is difficult to separate from the legitimate response of physicians to take more seriously the reporting of diagnoses when that report is tied to payment. Early studies of the potential impact of PPS were based on data in which diagnoses were not related to payment and hence were not always responsibly reported. Thus, some "coding creep" was expected as a legitimate part of the adjustment to the new system.

The PPS system was phased in over several years to allow hospitals time to adjust their behavior. Payments during this transition were a blend of the hospitals' 1982 costs (updated) and regional and national DRG rates. The actual phase-in took longer than the initially planned four-year period, finally shifting to full national rates in November 1987 (Russell 1989).

Since 1984, a number of ad hoc adjustments to PPS have been enacted by Congress, particularly with regard to geographic location and hospital characteristics. Usually these changes have shifted the categories to which certain hospitals are assigned or have added new dimensions to the payment system to compensate for what, at least politically, have been the perceived failings of the system in dealing with particular hospitals. Hospitals often argue that special circumstances cause them to be subject to higher costs than reflected in the DRG amounts.

Spirited lobbying and negotiation over these adjustments have kept Congress busy nearly every year since the passage of PPS. For example, hospitals that serve a disproportionate share of Medicare patients were granted additional payments beginning in 1986. In many cases, special treatment for some hospitals then lowers the payments made to others to keep budget neutrality in Medicare payments. This approach has effectively kept the hospital industry divided over the appropriate strategy for dealing with these changes.

Since passage of PPS, a consistent theme of federal budget reduction efforts has been to fund lower increases in payment rates to hospitals than that established in the original legislation. The PPS legislation called for an annual increase in payment levels, based on the prospective payment input price index (a "market basket" of hospital goods and services), adjustments for technological change, and an adjustment for changes in the mix of DRGs (a "case mix index") as a result of changes in coding and reporting accuracy (Ways and Means 1991).

The full update as calculated by the legislated formula has seldom been applied, however. Since 1985, the usual pattern has been for the administration to propose a very low update, which in turn is raised by Congress in its budget deliberations, reinstating some but not all of the increase that would have occurred if the original formula had been applied. These limits on the update modify the process established for the PPS system. They represent efforts to generate budget savings, but are also supported on the grounds that PPS began as a more generous system than was originally envisioned. As described next, hospitals, on average, did well financially during the early years of PPS. Nonetheless, hospitals often complain that although they are willing to abide by PPS, the reductions in the update penalize them for finding ways to cut costs. Together with PPS, the reduced updates resulted in a substantially lower rate of growth in hospital payments in the last half of the 1980s and early 1990s (figure 3.3).

The Immediate Response in Delivery of Care

The world did not stand still while PPS was being implemented. The healthcare environment for hospitals and other providers changed dramatically: developments in the practice of medicine affect what procedures are done in the hospital; other payers of healthcare have instituted their own strategies for holding down healthcare costs; states have revised their Medicaid payment methods; and many employers and insurers have sought discounts from hospitals as part of cost-containment efforts. Consequently, any analysis of trends in hospital care over the period captures what was happening in general and not just the specific impact of PPS.[12]

Nonetheless, some rather large jumps in key variables at the time PPS was implemented suggest that PPS has led to crucial changes in healthcare delivery and costs for patients, providers, and taxpayers. Two major changes in the way care is delivered occurred almost immediately: both lengths of stay per admission and number of admissions fell.

Hospitals moved swiftly to discharge their Medicare patients earlier. From 1983 to 1985, hospital stays for Medicare patients fell from 9.7 to 8.7 days, a decline of over 10 percent (NCHS 1991), accelerating an existing trend (see figure 3.4). Moreover, these reduced lengths of stay occurred for Medicare patients of all ages and across most DRG categories.

Admissions also dropped off sharply, as shown in table 3.3. Although shorter lengths of stay were anticipated as a response to the new incentives, the decline in admissions was unexpected. In fact, to help avoid the opposite problem of unnecessary hospitalization and to oversee the quality of care being delivered, a system of local Peer Review Organizations (PROs) was established simultaneously with PPS. It is plausible that the uncertainty caused by the new legislation and/or the scrutiny of the PROs over admissions did cause hospitals to reduce admissions. But it is also possible that PPS merely accelerated an existing trend toward performing simple surgical and diagnostic procedures on an outpatient basis. Since reimbursements were still based on the hospitals' costs in outpatient settings under PPS, hospitals did have incentives to shift care to that area. Whatever the reason, the combination of shorter stays and fewer admissions led to a dramatic decline in the total number of inpatient hospital days under Medicare through 1991. Since that time hospital admissions have been on the rise again (HCFA 1995).

These and other changes affected patients, hospitals, and federal spending in major ways. By changing so dramatically the way in which hospitals would be paid, all the interested parties faced new incentives and problems. The rest of this section examines those impacts on hospitals and the Medicare program, deferring to chapter 4 an assessment of the impact on Medicare beneficiaries.

Impacts on Hospitals

PPS provided hospitals with a number of opportunities to earn profits by reducing costs. But they could do so either at the expense of quality or by improving efficiency.

From the hospital's perspective, shorter periods of hospitalization *may* be associated with lower costs of care, but the savings may be considerably less than proportional. That is, if the number of tests and procedures remain the same, but are consolidated in fewer days of care, costs per case will not fall proportionately with shorter stays. And when shorter lengths of stay simply translate into more empty beds on average over the year, the fixed costs of the hospital will increase on a per case basis. Since the shorter length of stay occurred at the same time as a downturn in admissions, hospitals were faced with problems of excess capacity. Indeed, the American Hospital As-

Figure 3.4 AVERAGE LENGTH OF STAY IN NONFEDERAL SHORT-STAY HOSPITALS, 1980–93

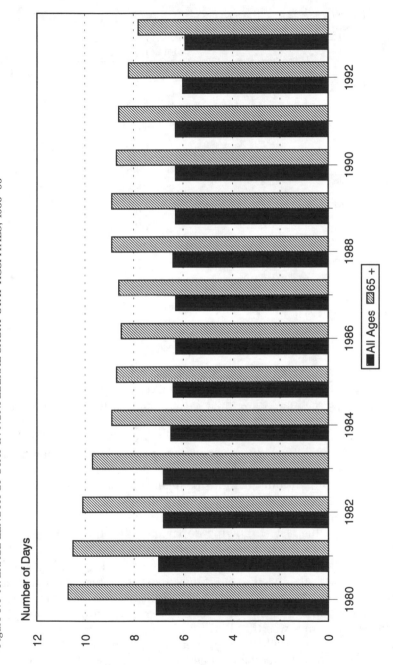

Source: NCHS (1995, 1991).

Table 3.3 RATE OF CHANGE IN HOSPITAL ADMISSIONS FOR MEDICARE
ENROLLEES, 1980–91

| Year | Community Hospitals | | |
	All (%)	Urban (%)	Rural (%)
1980	3.0	2.9	3.1
1981	0.8	3.5	−7.4
1982	−0.2	0.1	−0.9
1983	−0.6	0.7	−5.2
1984	−2.8	−2.0	−5.2
1985	−4.9	−3.9	−8.4
1986	−3.2	−2.3	−6.8
1987	−2.4	−1.6	−5.7
1988	−0.5	−0.1	−2.0
1989	−1.1	−0.7	−2.7
1990	0.2	0.4	−0.5
1991	−0.4	0.1	−2.4
Cumulative Change:			
1979–83	3.0	7.4	−10.3
1983–89	−13.9	−10.2	−27.3
1981–91	−14.7	−9.1	−33.7

Source: ProPAC (1993).

sociation has reported that in 1990, across all hospitals, one-third of
beds were empty, up sharply over 1980 (AHA 1991). For hospitals to
truly achieve savings, they must either do less for each patient or
provide the same services more efficiently (i.e., at less cost).

Hospitals did seek to reduce staff per patient—in particular, nursing staff (ProPAC 1991). But if the average patient is sicker than before
and more procedures are packed into fewer days, reducing the nursing
staff may, at some point, achieve cost reductions at the expense of
quality. The fact that other types of hospital personnel have not been
cut has fueled arguments about deteriorating quality of care. For example, among the fastest growing departments in hospitals over this
period were administrative services (ProPAC 1991). Some of this
growth no doubt reflects heavier burdens of dealing with the new
environment created by PPS, but it may also reflect reluctance to make
more sweeping changes. Hospitals have indeed been slow to institute
more fundamental reforms that alter the type of care delivered. For
example, one hope was that PPS would promote more emphasis on
cost-saving, as opposed to cost-increasing, technologies (Lave 1990).
This lack of innovative change has been a disappointment to some
early supporters of PPS. More recent studies of hospital behavior,

however, suggest the payment reforms or market pressures can lead to improved efficiency (Hadley et al. 1996).

The result of all of these changes was a steady decline in hospitals' Medicare operating margins in the first nine years after the introduction of PPS. These operating margins—defined as the difference between Medicare payments and Medicare-allowed inpatient operating costs—indicate how well Medicare covers the costs that hospitals incur in providing Medicare services. When PPS was introduced in 1983 and 1984, the level of payment to hospitals was quite generous, and hospitals' immediate response of reducing lengths of stay allowed many of them to do very well. Operating margins for Medicare averaged more than 14 percent in the first two years of the payment system. They declined thereafter, actually reaching a deficit in the seventh year of PPS (figure 3.5)[13] (ProPAC 1995a). Although the initial generosity of Medicare payments was to some extent intended to gain the acceptance of hospitals, as noted, the margins were even higher than many had anticipated.

Since then, legislative changes have held the update factors consistently below the market-basket adjustment that was supposed to protect hospitals from inflation and technological change. But large changes in the mix of DRGs over time toward higher weighted cases have led actual payments per discharge to grow more rapidly than indicated by the update factor.[14] Through the first seven years after PPS, payments to hospitals actually rose 69 percent. This trend suggests that cost-cutting efforts by Medicare have resulted in a reasonable balance of paying for costs. Critics of hospitals, however, argue that they have not had to make major adjustments to hold down their costs of care. Part of the reason for this may have been the ability of hospitals to tap into non-Medicare resources to protect their operating margins. But other payers are now also putting financial pressure on hospitals. This will produce an increasingly stringent test of the view that hospitals can cut costs through more increases in efficiency than they have implemented to date.

In any case, averages do not tell the whole story. Even in the early years of PPS when payments were more generous, individual hospitals varied substantially in their gains or losses in Medicare operating margins. Systematic variations also occur, causing certain types of hospitals to do better than others. As shown in table 3.4, major teaching hospitals and large urban disproportionate-share hospitals consistently have done much better, on average, than other hospitals (ProPAC 1995a). Since these types of facilities receive additional payments for each case, the findings are not surprising. Rural hospitals

Figure 3.5 AGGREGATE PPS OPERATING MARGINS

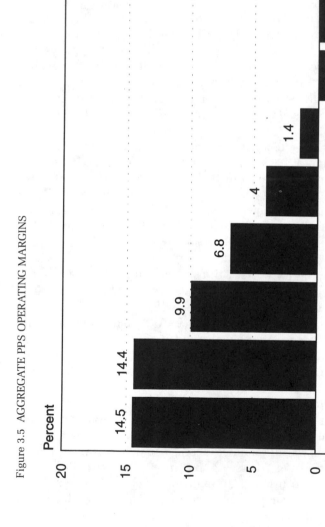

Source: ProPAC (1995a).

Table 3.4 DISTRIBUTION OF PPS OPERATING MARGINS, BY HOSPITAL GROUP, PPS 10

Hospital Group	Operating Margin by Percentile		
	25th (%)	Median (%)	75th (%)
All hospitals	−14.4	−1.7	8.6
Urban	−13.8	−1.9	8.2
Rural	−14.9	−1.3	9.1
Large urban	−13.4	.2	10.2
Other urban	−14.0	−3.3	6.1
Rural referral	−11.8	.3	7.6
Sole community	−14.1	1.2	12.3
Other rural	−15.9	−2.8	8.3
Major teaching	4.3	13.4	20.0
Other teaching	−9.5	.7	9.0
Nonteaching	−15.9	−3.1	7.7
Disproportionate Share:			
Large urban	−5.1	6.3	16.7
Other urban	−10.1	−.1	8.2
Rural	−12.2	1.7	12.1
Nondisproportionate share	−17.4	−4.2	6.4

Source: ProPAC (1995a).
Note: Excludes hospitals in Maryland. PPS 10 refers to the tenth year since the Prospective Payment System went into effect for hospitals.

with less than 50 beds have tended to have lower average Medicare operating margins than their large urban counterparts.

Within each type of hospital there are also big gainers and losers. Some major teaching hospitals have consistently low operating margins, whereas some small rural hospitals display consistently high operating margins. Indeed, a common complaint about Medicare PPS is this mismatch—that hospitals receiving the same payment levels may have varying costs that are not recognized by the system (ProPAC 1990).

How serious are the declines in Medicare operating margins? Clearly, Medicare margins have not fallen far enough to place most hospitals in overall financial distress. Rather, as noted, hospitals have cross-subsidized their operations from other more lucrative payers (i.e., private insurers). This safety valve of cost shifting effectively postpones the day of reckoning for hospitals, but it does not eliminate it. When their Medicare margins turn very negative and/or other payers do not provide enough revenue to maintain business as usual, hospitals will be forced to make major adjustments. This will come sooner for financially distressed hospitals. Indeed, the argument has been made (Sheingold 1986) that most of the cost-saving efforts to date under PPS have been made by hospitals in poor financial condition.

But this creates a dilemma. If hospitals respond only when they have to, more cuts may be necessary to induce those who are now shifting costs or who have positive margins to seek meaningful reforms in their operations. But further cuts may create intolerable pressures on those hospitals that have responded well to PPS but nonetheless have higher-than-average costs for legitimate but unrecognized reasons.

Impact on Medicare Administration

From the federal government's perspective, PPS has been very successful. It has achieved substantial reductions in benefit payments over time, not in absolute dollars, but in terms of what Medicare would otherwise have had to pay for care. This impact can be seen in the decline in the rate of growth of payments for inpatient services (figure 3.3).

One consequence of these changes was the steady outward progression of the date of projected exhaustion of the HI trust funds in the 1980s (see figure 3.6). In 1981, exhaustion was predicted by 1991. As indicated in previous chapters, policy changes have helped to steadily push off the date, so that by the 1991 trustees report, the date was 2005 (HI Trustees 1991). (The passage of PPS helped to protect the trust funds, and some of the low increases in hospital payments in later years—especially the updates for 1986 and 1990—were influential in postponing the date of exhaustion.)[15] However, between 1991 and 1992, a year when no legislative changes occurred, the date of exhaustion of the trust funds again slipped back to 2002 (HI Trustees 1992).

And since then, growth of home health and skilled nursing facility (SNF) services, which are also included in Part A of the program, has put further financial pressure on the system. These areas have not been subject to payment reforms and have become major contributors to Medicare's growth. The 1993 changes enacted for hospital services continued the trend of reducing payment updates, but even the large changes contained therein have not reversed the trend. Consequently, as shown earlier in figure 1.8, the estimated date of exhaustion is now 2001.

It is also possible that PPS may have been responsible for higher costs in home health and SNF by shifting costs to settings totally beyond the hospitals' doors. PPS is often cited as one reason for the

Figure 3.6 ESTIMATED BALANCE IN FEDERAL HOSPITAL INSURANCE TRUST FUND, SELECTED YEARS, 1982–2003

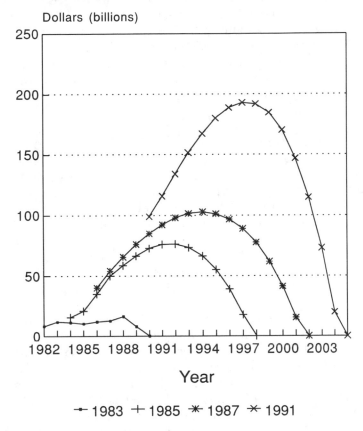

Year

━ 1983 ＋ 1985 ✳ 1987 ✳ 1991

Source: Board of Trustees, Federal Hospital Insurance Trust Fund, annual reports, selected years.

accelerated shift of treatment to standalone outpatient centers or physicians' offices. If so, some of the reduced spending on inpatient services will show up elsewhere, effectively offsetting the apparent cost-containment achievements of PPS. Shifts to skilled nursing facilities and to home health for postacute care would be captured by the trust fund projections in figure 3.6. But greater reliance on hospital outpatient services or physicians' offices is not captured by that indicator because these are Part B services. Between 1980 and 1988, hospital inpatient services grew 3 percent per year in real terms—that is, above the overall rate of inflation in the economy. The combined growth in hospital outpatient services, inpatient services, SNFs, and home health, in contrast to inpatient services alone, has been 4 percent per year—fully one-third higher. Not all of the additional growth in these services is attributable to PPS, nor would these offsets eliminate PPS savings. But PPS does provide evidence that savings may be less than indicated by focusing only on changes in hospital inpatient services. Decreases in cost in one part of the system have a nasty habit of popping up elsewhere.

Changes to Improve Hospital Payment

Few serious critics call for dismantling prospective payment; it is now an ingrained part of Medicare. Instead, there has been considerable interest in modifications to the PPS system that may strengthen it over time. One approach would be to reintroduce some hospital-specific costs into the formulas, recognizing that the payment factors in the current formula do not capture all the relevant variation (Hadley, Zuckerman, and Feder 1989; Lave 1990). This could provide protection for hospitals that have higher costs not accounted for by other adjustment factors and relieve one of the major criticisms leveled against PPS.[16]

Another proposal often discussed is to improve measures of illness severity to protect hospitals that treat sicker-than-average patients within each DRG. This solution focuses on one of the specific problems of PPS—the relative insensitivity of the system to differences across patients within a given DRG. If a hospital has an unusually high share of severely ill patients, it may effectively be penalized by PPS. Averaging across patients will not help if there is a persistent differential. Although the outlier policy was designed to ease this problem, it does not help if many patients are moderately sicker than average, as opposed to a few who are extreme cases.[17]

Others advocate further within-DRG adjustments or even alternatives to DRGs. Among the alternatives suggested are classifications systems that use objective, clinical data to generate more sensitive indicators (Office of Technology Assessment 1985; ProPAC 1986). But much of the attention directed to these types of adjustments to DRGs came in the mid-1980s, and interest since then has waned. Lave (1990) has also proposed "rebasing" the PPS system to capture the effects of changing costs of treatment across DRGs and increasing the number of adjustment factors. This would require reestimating the DRGs to better capture differences across hospitals in the costs of care provided to patients.

Some of the most recent proposals for reducing hospital spending have focused on the implicit subsidies to teaching hospitals for medical education and to hospitals that serve a disproportionate share of low-income and indigent patients. Phasing out or reducing such payments (or perhaps shifting them into other new programs) would lower Medicare's spending without reducing what is paid for basic hospital services.

All of these issues will become more urgent as greater efforts by the government to hold down costs put further pressures on hospitals. Unless new techniques refining DRGs that more effectively explain differences in costs can be developed, it makes sense to reintroduce some hospital-specific costs to the formula. Pressure needs to be applied to all hospitals to hold down costs, rather than just to those currently under financial stress. If we develop more confidence in the fairness of the payment mechanism, more stringent controls can be justified.

PHYSICIAN PAYMENT REFORM

From the outset, as already noted, Medicare sought to encourage physicians to participate. For this reason, initial payment levels were relatively generous and doctors were promised no restrictions as to the care they could provide. For the first 20 years of Medicare, physician reimbursement went largely unchanged. But physician payment growth became a major issue in the 1980s. Not only was growth high absolutely, but it was growing relative to hospital payments, which were moderating. Physicians also represent a target for cost-cutting efforts because of their high income levels and potential influence over the rest of healthcare spending.

Starting in 1984, payments were reduced through several mechanisms, including a freeze on how fast charges were allowed to grow. This fee freeze, first instituted on July 1, 1984, was viewed by many as a first step toward broader reform. This legislation permitted no increase in the "prevailing charge" for physicians—which acts as the absolute cap on Medicare allowed charges.[18] Since this represented a situation analogous to the TEFRA changes that helped push PPS for hospitals, many felt that reform could be hammered out before the freeze was lifted. But consensus remained elusive, and Congress failed to enact broader reform. After one further extension, the freeze was finally lifted in May 1986.[19] As figure 3.7 shows, despite the fee

Figure 3.7 ANNUAL RATES OF GROWTH IN MEDICARE PHYSICIAN PAYMENTS, 1976–1993

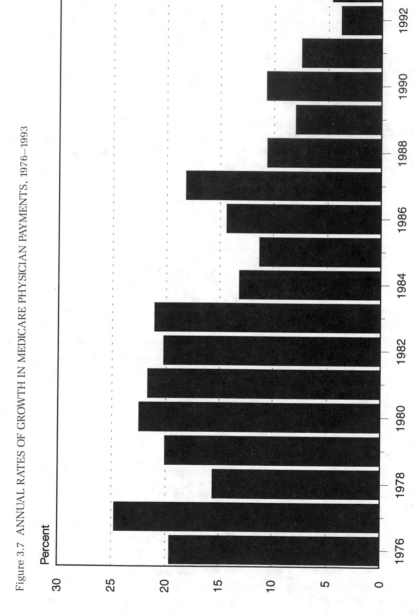

Source: Ways and Means (1994).

freeze, costs of the physician services portion of Part B continued to grow.

Many policymakers had long expressed doubts about Medicare's Part B payment structure, on the basis that it locked in historical inequities. These imbalances sent the wrong signals to physicians by paying relatively more for expensive, high-technology services while offering few incentives for careful geriatric assessments or other basic care. Further, payments in some rural areas of the country were viewed as too low, discouraging physicians from practicing in such areas. Finally, physician payments more generally varied enormously around the country and even within the same area for the same services—creating an extremely complex payment system that was not only difficult to manage but was also unable to provide appropriate incentives to physicians. Consequently, the old payment mechanism did not allow Congress or the Health Care Financing Administration (HCFA) to change incentives for physicians; a new mechanism was needed.

The desire to adopt reforms so as to control costs and eliminate payment inequities led to debate in the early 1980s about what approach to take. Some policymakers wanted the government to be able to set fees and streamline the payment process; others sought more dramatic schemes to pay physicians, not on a fee-for-service basis but, rather, on a flat amount per patient (referred to as "capitation" approaches). Often, this latter approach focused on using formal groups such as health maintenance organizations (HMOs) to oversee the volume of all service use (and not just physician services). The goal of simplifying the system so that it could be better controlled was also an important factor in the debate.

Fee reform may have stalled in the early 1980s, but recognition of the problem increased. In an attempt to speed the development of consensus on reform, Congress established a Physician Payment Review Commission (PPRC) in 1986 and charged it with hammering out the details of a reform package to propose to Congress and the Reagan administration. In March 1987, PPRC recommended a resource-based relative value scale (RBRVS) approach (PPRC 1987).[20] PPRC noted that this would not rule out further moves away from a fee-based system; rather, the fee schedule was emphasized as a necessary first step. The Reagan administration remained skeptical of relying only on a fee schedule, preferring more radical change to move away from a fee-for-service approach. Nonetheless, HCFA funded a major study of the RBRVS approach (Hsiao et al. 1988) that laid the groundwork for later physician payment reform that would indeed include a fee schedule in its structure.

Debate continued until 1989 when Congress, at the eleventh hour, passed the Medicare Fee Schedule as part of the Omnibus Budget Reconciliation Act of 1989 (OBRA89), based on the RBRVS approach. Like PPS, it was added to other more comprehensive legislation. The payment reform began on January 1, 1992, and, after a five-year transition, is now fully in place. The fee schedule does not reduce the overall level of payments to physicians, but it does substantially reduce payments for surgeries and procedures (which were deemed "overvalued") while increasing payments for basic office visits. As can be seen in figure 3.7, it has had a major impact on spending growth. As with the introduction of PPS, uncertainty surrounding a new system and an emphasis on finding ways to control spending may successfully affect the behavior of providers of care.

Implementation of the fee schedule has not been smooth, however. Doctors expressed outrage at a preemptive strike on reform in a 1990 budget agreement that essentially instituted some of the cuts in the "overvalued" procedures without offsetting increases in "undervalued" ones. But they exploded over an even more controversial move prior to the January 1, 1992, starting date—the release of proposed regulations for the fee schedule on June 5, 1991, in the *Federal Register*. Led by the AMA, doctors cried foul, not over the fee schedule but over the initial starting value (the "conversion factor"), which they felt violated the promise that the fee schedule be budget neutral. Two major sets of adjustments would effectively have resulted in a 16.5 percent cut in the conversion factor used to set fee levels.[21] The result would have been lower fees after the transition than physicians had expected to face. For example, HCFA calculated that an intermediate office visit for an established patient would rise only from $26 in 1991 before the fee schedule to $27 in 1992—not much of an increase for one of the fees that the schedule presumably sought to favor. There was thus little good news in fees to offset the bad news.

After much acrimony and threatened congressional intervention, HCFA produced its final regulations on November 11, 1991. The agency softened the cut in the conversion factor. As a consequence, that same intermediate office visit would now rise to $30 in 1992, rather than $27. The cuts were also reduced. For example, coronary artery bypass surgery would have fallen from $3,178 in 1991 to $2,726 in 1992 under the June rules, but only to $2,892 under the November rules. In retrospect some of these concerns proved correct; rates of growth in spending were lower than projected.

Details of the Medicare Fee Schedule

The general idea of a relative value scale had often been floated as a policy option in the debates over physician payment reform.[22] Policymakers are very attracted to the concept of directly establishing payment levels for various services, both absolutely and relative to each other. A relative value approach sets maximum levels of fees with the conscious goal of establishing justifiable differences across type of service. These relative values can then be translated into dollar fees at any absolute level desired.

The first sets of relative value scales in the United States were established using interviews with physicians to determine appropriate relationships among services. They represented standardization efforts more than attempts to rethink how fees are set. Early work by William Hsaio and William Stason (1979) moved the relative value scale in another direction, emphasizing a method for establishing values that was not dependent on existing fees or physicians' general perceptions regarding fees. They proposed the RBRVS, which would set the relative value units (RVUs) according to time and complexity of the service performed. The RVUs resulting from this study were at odds with earlier fee schedules and average reimbursement levels by various payers, weighting office visits more heavily relative to surgical procedures in the Hsaio-Stason approach.

The Hsaio-Stason findings appealed intuitively to many policymakers. First, they reflected a "scientific approach" that sought to establish RVUs objectively, rather than on the basis of historical precedent or individual physician judgment. Equally important, the approach suggested that high-technology procedures, which were growing rapidly and seemed well compensated, should fall relative to more basic services. If the findings of Hsaio and Stason had been in the opposite direction, it is likely that they would not have been nearly so well received. But this initial work was not undertaken in a vacuum. The policy "goals" of any new fee schedule were to raise fees for management and evaluation services and reduce those for surgery and other "overvalued" procedures. The Hsaio-Stason approach received support because it carried the assurance of leading in that direction.

The RBRVS approach also has many critics, who point out that prices in competitive markets reflect the value of services to consumers and not the costs of the inputs to produce the services (Hadley et al. 1986). Thus, the RBRVS may not produce relative values that reflect what individuals are actually willing to pay, and may lead to undesirable distortions in prices. These critics often favor instead a negotiated approach where the goals of the fee schedule and the market pressures can be reconciled directly.

The study commissioned by HCFA in anticipation of physician payment reform, noted earlier, was carried out by Hsaio and others at Harvard University, building on their earlier work. Published in 1988 (Hsaio et al. 1988), this work served as the basis for establishing the relative value units adopted by HCFA in 1991 (*Federal Register* 1991a).

The Harvard analysis used several techniques to devise RVUs. First, national surveys of 3,200 physicians and technical consulting groups representing 18 specialties were used to rate 23 key services in each specialty. These efforts resulted in within-specialty RVUs that then had to be compared across specialties. The next step was thus to "calibrate" these specialty-specific scales relative to each other, taking two specialties at a time. For a particular pair of specialties, several key services in each specialty were compared by expert panels to provide rankings that could link the specialty-specific scales.[23] Then the whole package was combined. This yielded a set of key RVUs that then served as the basis for establishing rankings for other services. Within a specialty, existing charges for groups of services were used to set the final RVUs.[24]

The process was expensive and time-consuming, representing a careful effort to establish an objective measure of "value." However, it is certainly not perfect science, nor did it satisfy everyone. The cross-specialty linkages were subject to considerable debate, and many physicians believed their own services were ranked too low. In general, however, there was considerable acceptance of the study's methodology, and the findings again had intuitive appeal. Physicians' groups, who viewed some type of reform as inevitable, generally agreed to this type of approach.

The RBRVS constitutes only one of three major parts of the Medicare Fee Schedule. The first part is a fee schedule that establishes "national uniform relative values for all physicians' services" that are the sum of the RVUs that reflect physician work, practice expenses (net of physician liability insurance), and the cost of professional liability insurance. These national relative values are then modified by a geographic adjustment factor. Finally, a conversion factor is applied to the adjusted RVUs to achieve dollar values for the fees. Unlike the earlier RBRVS by Hsaio and Stason, the Medicare Fee Schedule has no adjustments for specialty per se. Consequently, specialists who concentrate on surgeries or procedures that were substantially cut will face large reductions in Medicare services.

HCFA turned to Urban Institute studies by Stephen Zuckerman, W. Pete Welch, and Gregory Pope (1990) in developing a geographic adjustment factor for the Medicare Fee Schedule. The geographic practice cost index (GPCI) proposed by these authors represents an effort to measure the relative costs of inputs used in practices across the United States. In many cases, data on the relevant price variation do not routinely exist, and proxy data are needed to derive the index. For example, it is very difficult to obtain information on office rents in some areas of the country, necessitating that apartment rent differences be included as a proxy. Although the original data on the GPCI included professional liability expenses (for malpractice), these were specifically established as a separate factor in the legislation, recognizing that these adjustments were likely to be subject to further change in the future and indeed, HCFA is currently proceeding on redesigning the GPCI.

Another element of physician payment reform consists of volume performance standards (VPS), designed to create incentives to moderate the rate of growth in expenditures for physicians' services. These standards are then used by Congress in setting the rate of growth of physician payments each year. If Congress fails to act on a specific rate, a default formula dictates the level of payment. Essentially the formula creates a penalty that varies in inverse relation to the rate of growth in the volume of services over the previous five years that is not attributable to enrollee growth, regulation, or legislation. At present, there are two VPS calculations: one for surgery and one for nonsurgery. Each is applied on a national level. Early critics contended that this scale was too broad to have the desired effect on physician behavior and that the standards would end up penalizing physicians who are not gaming the system. But policy proposals have moved in the opposite direction—seeking to create one uniform national standard.

Finally, the reform legislation limited the ability of physicians to bill their patients above Medicare's fees ("extra billing"). This was a compromise between consumer groups who wanted to require Medicare fees to represent payment in full and physicians who opposed all such limits. Limits on extra billing protect the financial resources of the elderly and those with disabilities, but also may result in restrictions on access to care if physicians decline to take on Medicare patients as a result. Physicians argued that without such opportunities for additional billing, fees would be undesirably restrictive, preventing differences across physicians on the basis of the quality of care, for example. In the end, the limits adopted were quite stringent.

Physicians who decline to "accept assignment" (see note 19) are able to bill only about 10 percent above the fee levels.[25] Before these limits were imposed, beneficiaries often faced balanced billing amounts equal to or higher than their copayments.

The Impact of the Fee Schedule

One objective *not* achieved by the fee schedule is simplicity. With over 7,000 codes and 233 geographic areas, the MFS consists of thousands of separate fees, although it does represent some simplification over the old system. While it is a challenge for physicians to keep track of their own fees, at least now they can be known in advance. The regulations of this complicated system took up 317 pages in the *Federal Register* (1991a). And changes in the fee schedule have continued to be made during the transition process.

As intended, the Medicare Fee Schedule has shifted Medicare payments from procedural services toward evaluation and management services (table 3.5). Payments for primary care services grew at an average annual rate of 6.9 percent between 1992 and 1995, and other evaluation and management services rose at an annual rate of 5.4 percent over the same period. In contrast, payments for surgical services grew at an average of only 2.8 percent and other nonsurgical service payment growth was negative. Almost certainly as a result of the change, primary care delivery has increased as a proportion of allowed charges (HCFA 1995).

Volume and intensity growth has also declined since the late 1980s. Between 1991 and 1993, estimated Medicare expenditure growth on physician services averaged 3.8 percent, below the performance standard guidelines (PPRC 1996). As a consequence, no downward adjustments were made in the conversion factors. Across the 1992 to 1995 period, growth rates in service volume depended on type of service, with some of the new technologies (such as magnetic resonance imaging and arthroscopy) and emergency room visits above 10 percent on an annual basis and surgical procedures showing considerably slower growth (table 3.5).

The slow growth in the volume of surgical services is particularly interesting. Different volume performance standards were adopted in the Medicare Fee Schedule on the assumption that surgical procedures might grow rapidly and be in need of tighter controls. But since the opposite has happened, updates in surgical versus primary care fees have not increased the incentive to deliver primary care services as was initially anticipated.

Table 3.5 CHANGE IN PAYMENT AND USE PER BENEFICIARY FOR SELECTED
SERVICES, 1992–1995

Type of Service	Annual Percentage Change			Percentage of 1995 Physician Services Outlay
	Payment per Service	Volume[a]	Count of Services[b]	
All Services	2.8	5.1	4.8	100.0
Primary Care Services	6.9	5.1	4.3	21.2
Office and other outpatient visits	6.2	4.0	3.7	16.4
Emergency department	9.0	10.4	8.6	2.5
Nursing facility/rest home	10.8	8.7	7.1	1.9
Home visits	10.7	5.5	4.9	0.2
Other Evaluation and Management Services	5.4	6.0	3.5	17.5
Surgical Services	2.8	3.3	6.8	21.9
Cataract lens replacement	− 1.1	− 0.3	− 0.3	3.3
Joint prosthesis	2.2	6.0	5.5	1.4
Coronary artery bypass graft	2.6	6.5	7.4	1.3
Transurethral prostate surgery	5.6	− 11.2	− 10.9	0.4
Arthroscopy	1.6	8.6	8.4	0.2
Other Nonsurgical Services	− 0.2	5.8	5.0	39.3
Diagnostic radiology, other	0.2	1.4	1.8	3.2
Echocardiograms	− 5.1	14.4	14.8	1.9
CAT scans	− 0.1	4.0	5.1	1.5
Colorectal endoscopy	− 0.8	3.3	− 1.3	1.4
Magnetic resonance imaging	1.6	12.0	12.4	1.0
Angioplasty	− 6.5	11.6	11.5	0.6
Mammography	1.1	− 0.7	1.8	0.4

Source: PPRC (1996).
a. Measures change in outlays if prices were frozen (volume and intensity).
b. Measures change in the number of services only.

Finally, as will be discussed further in the next chapter, access to
physician care by beneficiaries has not suffered overall. To some extent, this may have been aided by the narrowing gap between Medicare
and private physician fees in the 1990s (Miller, Zuckerman, and Gates
1993). In 1996, Medicare is projected to pay about 71 percent of private
sector rates on average (PPRC 1996). This reflects changes going on in
the private sector as well as Medicare changes, but the result is that
Medicare is less at a disadvantage in its payments to physicians than
it used to be, taking pressure off Medicare to take additional steps to
ensure that beneficiaries are not denied access.

OTHER PROVIDER CHANGES

Although most of the cost-containment attention has been directed at inpatient hospital and physician services, which represent the biggest shares of Medicare, other areas have also been subject to the budget ax. Indeed, the effort has been so extensive that micromanagement of budget cutting reached new heights in the 1990 budget deal. To achieve $43 billion in five-year savings, almost no part of Medicare remained unscathed. For example, payments for prosthetic devices were frozen, further restrictions were added to the coverage of seat-lift chairs and power scooters, and reductions were made in laboratory fees. These changes produced only a tiny portion of the $43 billion, but spread the pain across many providers. And again in 1993, a broad range of changes affected nearly all parts of Medicare.

During the 1980s, additional areas were subject to substantial cost-saving efforts. For example, home health and skilled nursing care benefits were constrained by interpretation of regulations rather than from legislative changes. Savings in other areas have been a bit more elusive. Outpatient hospital services, which have grown enormously, received considerable attention and some cost cutting, but major policy change has not been seen in that area. Payment policy for outpatient services remains a hodgepodge of ad hoc adjustments (Sulvetta 1992), with scheduled payment reform delayed several times. Congress first mandated recommendations from HCFA by April 1989 (Ways and Means 1989). HCFA is still working on its final recommendations. When those changes come they are likely to result in a PPS-type system. Limited efforts have also focused on fraud and abuse— such as attention to physician referrals to laboratories or testing facilities in which they have a financial stake.

Home Health Services

Home health under Medicare has always been limited to "skilled" care, thereby restricting its size. Nonetheless, the benefit has undergone a number of "phases." In the early years of the program, growth was relatively restricted, in large part by limits on the number of services and the existence of cost sharing. Those restrictions were fully lifted by 1980, resulting in a rapid rate of growth in the benefit. A period of extremely tight regulatory control then followed in the mid-1980s, with a subsequent easing of restrictions after an important court case (discussed later in this section) at the end of the decade.

Since 1989, the rate of growth of spending on these benefits has taken off (figure 3.8).

Home health services represent a medical benefit to which enrollees are eligible if they are under the care of a physician, confined to home, and need skilled nursing services on an intermittent basis. Coverage is also available for those who need physical or speech therapy (and at least earlier have met the other criteria). The coinsurance requirement for home health was removed in 1972, and further liberalization in 1980 eliminated the deductible, the 100-day limit, and the prior hospitalization requirement. This means that nearly all home health services effectively were shifted to Part A.[26] In addition, in 1980, proprietary agencies were permitted to operate without licensing requirements, leading to a rapid expansion in the supply of home health services—and likely having the greatest impact on use of services (Kenney 1990).

Concern about rates of growth in reimbursement for home health in excess of 25 percent a year between 1980 and 1983 led HCFA to closely scrutinize intermediaries' adherence to the eligibility requirements and types of services received. HCFA clamped down on activities and instructed its intermediaries to closely examine claims. Denial rates increased (Leader 1988) and the rate of growth of reimbursements slowed noticeably, at a time when the introduction of PPS would have been expected to accelerate growth. By 1986, the rate of growth in reimbursements slowed to 1.1 percent, and actually declined in 1987 (Ways and Means 1991).

The regulatory strategy to hold down costs proved very effective. In 1984, HCFA issued new guidelines to the fiscal intermediaries regarding the interpretation of the part-time and intermittent requirements. The 1984 guidelines required that an otherwise eligible individual would qualify for the benefit only if the care were both part-time (less than eight hours per day) and intermittent (four or fewer days per week). Eligibility also required that the individual be homebound. This meant a virtual Catch 22, where the individual had to be so incapacitated as to be unable to operate outside the home, but well enough to need only part-time care.

Since that time, an important lawsuit, *Duggan v. Bowen*, has helped to ease these requirements substantially.[27] Beginning in July 1989, the definitions of medical necessity changed, the definition of intermittency was relaxed, and the guidelines to intermediaries were rewritten to establish more consistent treatment. The impact has been to allow an enormous expansion of services beginning in 1989, as indicated by figure 3.8.

Figure 3.8 BENEFIT PAYMENTS UNDER MEDICARE PART A: 1975–93

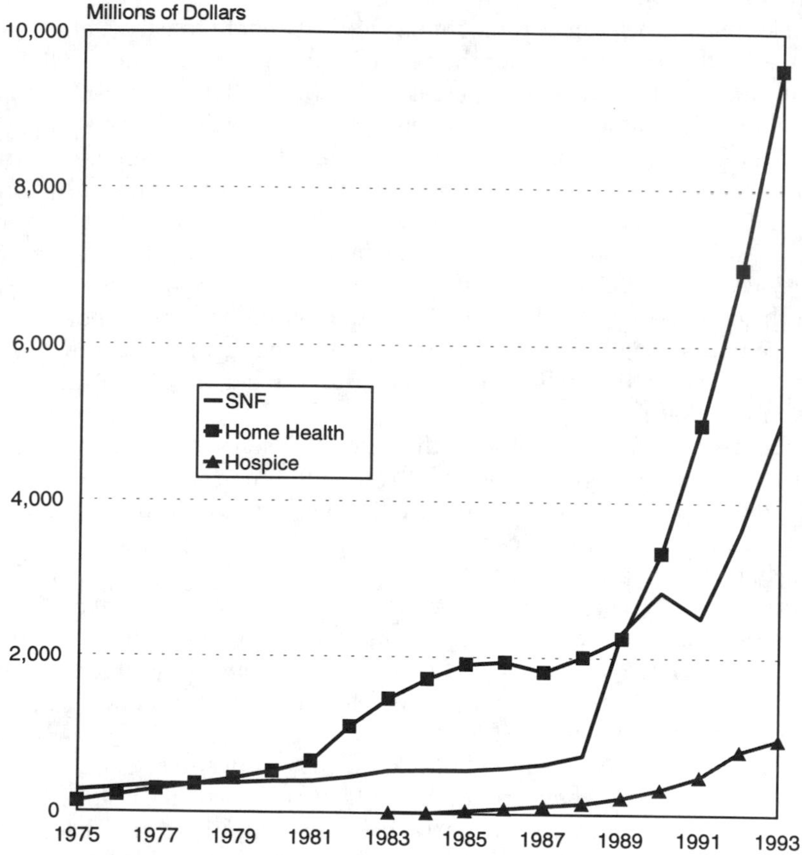

Source: Ways and Means (1994).

The period of strong cost containment in home health of the 1980s was followed by rapid growth on several fronts. Between 1989 and 1994, Medicare spending on home health increased fivefold and now accounts for 8 percent of all Medicare spending. Rates of growth over this period averaged almost 37 percent annually—a rate of growth more than three times that of the rest of the Medicare program. Most of this expansion has occurred in the use of services rather than in payment levels. Between 1988 and 1994, the proportion of beneficiaries receiving home health services nearly doubled and the average number of visits per user almost tripled (Kenney and Moon 1996).

And much of this growth in visits has occurred for persons receiving 100 or more visits, shifting this service more toward a long-term care benefit. Many of these long-term users of home health are getting home health aide visits, which are less-skilled services. Such visits are also likely to be lucrative for home health agencies since they do not require nearly the same skill levels in providing care but are still highly compensated by Medicare. But some home health care remains a brief recovery ("subacute") service: about a quarter of all users have nine or fewer visits, usually after a hospital stay. Home health benefits seem to be serving a dual purpose, caring for both the short- and long-term needs of beneficiaries.

The number of agencies providing services has also expanded by 30 percent, with particularly strong growth in the number of proprietary agencies. This is also changing the character of the home health benefit, which used to be dominated by the Visiting Nurse Association and other nonprofit providers of service. The new proprietary agencies are also more likely to concentrate on less-skilled services.

The changing home health benefit under Medicare is thus an area where little has been done in recent years to contain costs and where, appropriately, future attention is likely to focus. Legislation to reduce spending on Medicare in 1993 placed a freeze on updating the maximum amount that could be paid per home health visit. This stopgap measure produced savings, but does not take the place of more comprehensive reform because it is service use where cost increases are centered and where at least some controls are needed. Finding appropriate ways to implement such controls will be challenging, however, because the Medicare home health benefit is both serving a range of very different needs and changing rapidly over time.

Skilled Nursing Facility Care

Like home health, skilled nursing facility (SNF) care has always been constrained by its definition. SNF benefits are restricted to enrollees who have had a three-day prior hospital stay and who need skilled nursing or rehabilitation services. In 1969, they were limited to those on a course of recovery. These limitations restrict the number of persons eligible and ensured that Medicare never became a substantial provider of long-term care services (Smits, Feder, and Scanlon 1982). In addition, until the late 1980s intermediaries had regulatory discretion over what conditions qualified for SNF reimbursement and the duration of benefits, interpretations that varied widely across the United States (Liu and Kenney 1991). Earlier studies criticized the arbitrary and after-the-fact rulings about coverage that discouraged nursing home participation (Smits et al. 1982). Nonetheless, they represented an important cost constraint on SNF care that seems to have become more important during the mid-1980s, when PPS was leading to earlier hospital discharges than ever before. Perhaps the most crucial cost-control force, however, has been the relatively low reimbursement rates under Medicare.

In the 1980s, cost-sharing requirements became more severe. The level of SNF cost sharing (assessed against days 21 through 100) is tied to the hospital deductible, which rose rapidly in the 1980s and outpaced the growth in the costs of SNF care. In fact, at one-eighth of the hospital deductible, the SNF cost sharing turns out to be nearly as high as the daily payment to some providers of SNF care. Consequently, for many beneficiaries, the SNF benefit essentially became only a 20-day benefit (Liu and Kenney 1991), with other private arrangements after that. This was yet another force keeping growth in the SNF benefit down without formal policy change (see figure 3.8).

The situation changed substantially in April 1988, when a legal ruling established more uniform coverage guidelines, taking away one of the barriers to receiving care. Much of the discretion employed by intermediaries in interpreting what services were covered was eliminated. Consequently, heavy-care patients such as those requiring tube feeding became eligible for the first time (Liu and Kenney 1991). SNF reimbursements took a sharp upward jump, a movement that continued in 1989 with the addition of benefits from the Medicare Catastrophic Coverage Act (described in chapter 5). The SNF expansions from that legislation were later repealed, but SNF use did not return to its earlier levels of low growth, due at least in part to the large numbers of nursing facilities that geared up to serve Medicare patients in 1989. Expenditures grew from $2.5 billion in 1990 to $9.0 billion in 1995, more than tripling in five years. Disproportionately higher growth in this service area is expected to continue, making it another likely candidate for further cost-containment efforts (Moon et al. 1995).

HEALTH MAINTENANCE ORGANIZATIONS

Since 1985, Medicare has allowed health maintenance organizations (HMOs) to contract with the government to serve beneficiaries in exchange for a set monthly payment.[28] HMOs then take on the risk of providing the full range of Medicare benefits to those who enroll. This option, designed to allow Medicare to take advantage of managed care, promises to control costs by overseeing the full range of services delivered. It also makes the costs to Medicare more predictable, because HMOs charge a fixed payment per beneficiary.

Enrollment in HMOs initially grew rapidly, albeit from a very small base. In 1985, only 3.6 percent of Medicare beneficiaries were enrolled in some type of HMO (HCFA 1995). By 1987, enrollment grew by more than 50 percent. After that it leveled off and enrollment only reached 2 million by 1991 (see table 3.6). Since that time, the numbers of beneficiaries signing up for HMOs has increased dramatically. By the end of 1995, 3.8 million were enrolled. However, enrollment remains spotty, with large shares of enrollees signing up in Southern California, Florida, Oregon, and New York, while vast parts of the country have little or no Medicare HMO penetration. And, Medicare HMO enrollment continues to lag behind the move toward managed care for the nonelderly population.

Controversy exists over whether the HMO program has generated any savings for Medicare. The essential step in generating savings is determining how to pay HMOs—a critical factor in ensuring that competition among plans occurs fairly. Medicare bases its payment on an estimate of the average amount it would have spent on beneficiaries if they had remained in the traditional fee-for-service program. The amount (referred to as the adjusted average per capita cost or AAPCC) is calculated for each county in the United States and reflects differences by age, gender, and whether the beneficiary is institutionalized. Medicare then pays 95 percent of that amount in order to generate savings for the program. But savings only result if the AAPCC is less than what those enrolling would otherwise have cost Medicare.

Whether this is the case has been called into question because of findings suggesting that healthier-than-average beneficiaries—or at

Table 3.6 MEDICARE BENEFICIARIES ENROLLED IN HMOs

Year	Number in HMOs	Percent of Total Medicare Population
1985	1,121	3.6%
1987	1,735	5.4
1989	1,787	5.3
1991	2,025	5.8
1993	2,482	6.8
1995	3,807	10.1

Source: HCFA (1995).

least those who use less than average numbers of health services—
are more likely to enroll. If HMOs do indeed attract Medicare beneficiaries selectively—seeking beneficiaries whose average costs will
be lower than Medicare's per capita payment because they are low-
risk patients—then the HMO program may be more expensive for
Medicare as a whole (Langwell and Hadley 1989). The most comprehensive study to date found that Medicare beneficiaries enrolled in
HMOs only cost about 89 percent of the average, suggesting that Medicare was paying more to HMOs than they were spending on care
(Brown et al. 1993). Since that study was conducted, Medicare HMO
enrollments have increased substantially and things may have
changed. A more recent but considerably less comprehensive study
suggests less selection (Rodgers and Smith 1996).

Whatever the case concerning selection and current HMO enrollment, however, the AAPCC is not a very satisfactory mechanism for
establishing payment levels. Work is underway to improve upon this
methodology. As managed care plans expand and as proposals to
promote them further are offered, this will be an important element
in determining whether options for choosing private plans truly act
as a means of cost savings under Medicare.

CONCLUSIONS

Overall, Medicare's achievements in cost containment have been remarkable. At a time when many payers of healthcare—insurers and
employers—complained about costs but demonstrated little inclina-
tion to experiment with dramatic solutions, Medicare forged ahead.
Prodded by Congress, HCFA undertook sweeping changes affecting
payments for hospitals and physicians. And, although there have certainly been problems, the innovations offered by the government have
both held down costs and served as a model for others to emulate and
build upon. From 1985 through 1992 rates of growth in Medicare
spending were actually below those of private insurers on a per capita
basis (Moon and Zuckerman 1996).

For hospitals, PPS helped to bring down the growth in costs of
healthcare for the Medicare program and, at least for innovative hospitals, provides incentives for improved efficiency. Perhaps the greatest failing of PPS is its inability to account for some legitimate differences in costs that lead to overly generous payments for some
hospitals and insufficient levels for others. Further tinkering and ad-

justment of the system will undoubtedly continue. But it is unlikely that Medicare will reject the PPS system and either return to the old ways or seek some radically different approach. Some concerns about quality (discussed in chapter 4) also warrant continued monitoring of the system.

For physicians, payment reform has represented a considerable improvement over the previous payment scheme. The tools are at hand to discipline both price and volume growth and both these controls seem to be working. That other payers have adopted the RBRVS approach provides a further sign of its success.

This era of cost control is not over, however. The 1990s have seen fewer changes thus far, but a number of areas are ripe for further reform. Payment system reforms for home health, skilled nursing care, and outpatient hospital services have been proposed and although not yet enacted, these areas will undoubtedly be subject to legislation in the near future. The role of private plans—either HMOs or a broader collection of choices—as an alternative to traditional Medicare will become ever more important as well.

Notes

1. The picture would likely change if hospital *outpatient* services were included, since much of the drop in hospital use reflected a move to outpatient services. In addition, after 1989, if home health and skilled nursing costs were separated from hospital care, very different patterns would emerge. Home health and skilled nursing care have been growing at double digit rates.

2. Once Medicare payment rates differ from the general rate of price increases in the economy, the medical price index does not neatly separate price and volume differences. Care should thus be taken in assuming that use of services grew little after 1982, as implied by figure 3.1.

3. The MEI establishes the limit on the yearly increase in physicians' prevailing charges under Medicare. Prevailing charges reflect the 75th percentile of all physician charges for that particular service in a given area. Since not all physicians' bills are as high as the prevailing charges in an area, this is not an absolute cap, however.

4. The limits now applied to ancillary departments and special care units, and for each case, the hospital would get its target or 120 percent of the average cost for similar hospitals, whichever was lower.

5. Hospitals with costs below both sets of limits could keep one-half of the difference between their costs and the TEFRA limits.

6. A unique DRG is assigned to a patient depending upon diagnosis at admission and the type of treatment received (i.e., whether surgery was performed). Diagnoses and procedures are identified by codes defined in the International Classification of Diseases

(referred to as ICD-9 codes). This system had been developed at Yale University and was used in the state of New Jersey. However, no one had studied applications of DRGs specifically for aged and disabled persons.

7. In the early years of PPS, "age 70 or over" was used as a proxy to capture more expensive cases; that has now been replaced by "complicating condition" (Lave 1990).

8. Outliers are those patients whose length of stay in the hospital or whose costs of care are way above the average for other patients in the same DRG. Outlier limits are established for each DRG and apply to only a small fraction of patients (about 5 percent).

9. Weights are updated annually to reflect changing relative costs. New procedures are added occasionally; there are now 490 DRGs. Moreover, as patterns of care or treatments change, the weights for the DRGs also change. This "recalibration" attempts to keep DRGs current with technology and other factors that affect the costs of hospital care. Since 1989, new DRGs have joined the top ten, including chronic obstructive pulmonary disease, psychoses, and respiratory infections, while others have cycled off.

10. When PPS was passed, capital costs—those associated with building or modifying facilities and purchasing equipment—were excluded from the calculation of other costs. Such costs vary substantially from year to year and offer major challenges for payment design. Rather than trying to design that part of PPS at time of passage, payment policy retained capital payments as a "pass through" in the formula. Payments used the pre-PPS methodology and were added to a hospital's PPS payment each year. Congress instructed the U.S. Department of Health and Human Services to devise a prospective payment scheme for capital costs. HCFA has adopted regulations for capital payments that are essentially comparable to the methodology used for establishing PPS payments. The rates are fully prospective and not related to actual spending levels by hospitals. And like PPS, there are special provisions and exceptions for certain types of hospitals. A longer, 10-year transition to this system has been proposed, in recognition that hospitals make decisions regarding capital investments well in advance. A 1996 change also alters the update method to directly establish payment growth.

11. These issues are discussed in chapter 4.

12. Some studies were able to examine the staggered transition to PPS to analyze its impact on hospital care. These have suggested that PPS was indeed important (Coulam and Gaumer 1991). In addition, a few states received waivers that allowed them to avoid using the PPS system. Some studies have used these states' experiences as controls for examining PPS impact, although these waivered states certainly do not constitute a random control group.

13. The Prospective Payment Assessment Commission (ProPAC) estimates operating margins according to time elapsed since the beginning of the PPS for each hospital. Since hospitals vary in their fiscal years, they entered the system at differing dates in 1983 and 1984. PPS year six would be approximately 1990.

14. Some of this discrepancy is accounted for by real increases in the severity of cases and some is an artifact of DRG "code creep."

15. Between 1975 and 1980, hospital inpatient services per enrollee grew 7 percent annually after adjusting for general inflation (CBO 1991). That growth rate declined to 3.4 percent for the 1980 to 1990 period. Actual spending in 1990 was only 71 percent of what it would have been if the 1975 to 1980 trend of spending had continued in the 1980s. However, although PPS and the scrutiny of the PROs may account for some of that trend, admission rates for persons of all ages also fell over this period, likely

reflecting changes in the ways we use hospitals in the United States, more reliance on outpatient services, and perhaps even changes in the overall health of our citizens.

16. To guard against returning payment to a cost-plus environment, however, the cost calculations could use a base year trended forward using an index independent of behavior. This would be similar to the methodology employed under TEFRA.

17. Implicitly, adjustments for disproportionate-share and teaching hospitals have also sought to offer such protections, but these are proxy measures targeting hospitals likely to have such patients. Disproportionate-share hospitals refer to those with an unusually high proportion of Medicare and Medicaid patients. Teaching hospitals train a substantial share of medical interns and residents. Both types of hospitals, it is argued, are likely to have sicker patients or patients with other complicating conditions that make them more expensive to treat. These approaches do not address problems of higher costs for hospitals that do not fit into a protected category, however.

18. Physicians whose charges were below the prevailing rate could receive higher payments over this period until they hit the prevailing cap.

19. Actually, the freeze was lifted only for those physicians who agreed to "accept assignment" for all their Medicare patients (i.e., "participating" physicians who agreed to bill Medicare directly rather than demanding that their patients pay in full at the time of service). Physicians who did not agree to accept assignment for all patients remained under the freeze until January 1, 1987.

20. This approach would set fees for physicians on the basis of physician time and practice costs necessary to perform the service.

21. The more controversial of the reasons for these adjustments was HCFA's decision to anticipate a likely increase in the volume of services by reducing the conversion factor by 10.5 percent. This adjustment was disputed on several grounds, especially the assumption that physicians would game the system. It thus condemned them before the fact. The second reason for the adjustment was a technical issue related to the transition rules established by Congress.

22. Using a fee schedule was also debated. One camp argued for negotiated fees, to be decided after tough bargaining between the government and groups representing physicians. Others advocated relative value scales that would establish new fees based on time spent and/or intensity of effort. Lack of consensus on appropriate strategies for change also slowed efforts to reform Medicare payment policy (Hadley et al. 1986).

23. These panels consisted of but a small number of physicians, an aspect of the Harvard study (Hsaio et al. 1988) that has been criticized.

24. Since then, further analysis has been undertaken by the Harvard researchers to analyze more procedures and more specialties. Moreover, the legislation adopting the Medical Fee Schedule also drew on modifications in the methodology provided by the PPRC (1989).

25. The actual limit is 15 percent, but nonparticipating physicians are paid only 95 percent of the fee level.

26. Originally, the benefit was covered under Part A for patients who had either been hospitalized or admitted to a skilled nursing facility for at least three days, or under Part B for patients without prior hospital or SNF admissions. Once benefits were exhausted under Part A (after 100 days per spell of illness), they were available under Part B, but were subject to the Part B deductible and coinsurance.

27. *Duggan v. Bowen*, designed to clarify home health eligibility criteria, was settled out of court when HCFA agreed to make certain changes (Dubay, Kenney, Liu, and Moon 1991).

28. Before 1985, beneficiaries were able to enroll in some HMOs on a cost basis.

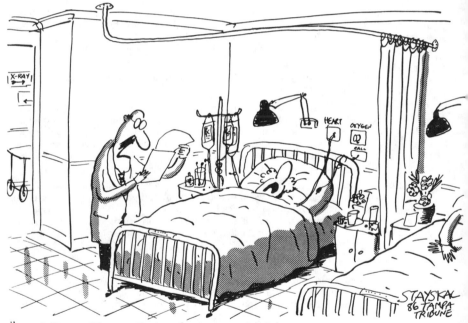

"YOUR BLOOD PRESSURE AND TEMPERATURE ARE WAY UP, BUT YOUR MEDICARE COVERAGE IS WAY DOWN. LOOKS AS IF YOU CAN GO HOME TODAY, MRS. FITCH!"

Chapter Four

CONTAINING COSTS: IMPACTS ON BENEFICIARIES

Cost-containment efforts affect beneficiaries directly by raising what they are required to pay (cost sharing) and indirectly through requirements on hospitals, doctors, and other healthcare providers. Direct burdens come in the form of increased cost sharing, Part B premiums, and out-of-pocket expenses on uncovered services. They change not only as a result of direct policy change but also simply as a function of changes in overall spending on Medicare-covered services. In 1995, total spending on benefits covered by Medicare amounted to $5,561 for the average beneficiary. Of that total, beneficiaries paid $1,261 on average in required cost sharing and Part B premiums—almost one-quarter (23 percent) of the costs of Medicare-covered services (see figure 4.1). Noncovered acute-care services raise the beneficiary share of total healthcare costs to about 30 percent of all acute-care services.

This 30 percent still does not capture the entire beneficiary burden, however, because it does not include the indirect effects on beneficiaries from policy changes that affect provider behavior. These lead to changes in the healthcare market that ultimately affect how and how much healthcare is delivered. Shorter hospital stays in response to Medicare's hospital PPS, for example, have likely led beneficiaries to substitute other types of services, such as homemaker aides. Such services are not usually covered by Medicare but are also not included in the 30 percent figure because they are not acute-care services. Beneficiaries also clearly suffer from reductions in care that could have extended life or improved its quality. And declines in the quality of care that may result from cost containment represent even less tangible, but no less important, beneficiary burdens.

Most of the major changes since 1980 have been in provider reimbursement. This chapter begins with a discussion of the more minor changes in beneficiary cost sharing. It then proceeds to examine indirect changes in beneficiary burden from the implementation of PPS on hospitals, a major issue, and ends with a focus on quality of care.

Figure 4.1 PER CAPITA MEDICARE EXPENDITURES: FEDERAL SHARE AND
BENEFICIARY LIABILITY, ADJUSTED FOR INFLATION

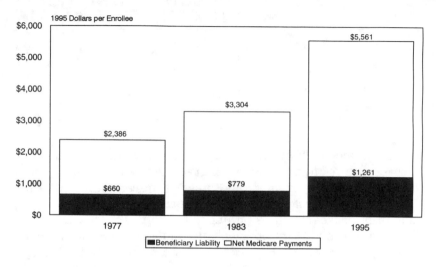

Source: HCFA (1995); U.S. Bureau of the Census (1996).

DIRECT CHANGES IN BENEFICIARY COST SHARING

Legislative changes in the 1980s altered the degree to which beneficiaries are required to pay additional shares of the costs of their Medicare-covered acute care. Although none of these increases individually proved very significant, when added together they generated
substantial savings to the Medicare program and added noticeably to
enrollees' average liabilities. In every budget submission by Presidents
Reagan and Bush, proposed cuts in Medicare affecting beneficiaries
have constituted a substantial share of the domestic budget reduction
agenda. In turn, Congress included beneficiaries in each of the major
budget reduction reconciliation acts of the 1980s, although generally
to a lesser degree than the administration advocated. Thus, the elderly
and disabled populations were not immune to the budget cutting of
the 1980s.

Sources of Higher Beneficiary Burdens

The largest Medicare cuts in the first budget that was passed during the Reagan administration (1981) occurred in beneficiary cost sharing. That budget reconciliation act raised the deductible amounts for both parts of Medicare. The deductible under Part B rose from $60 to $75— a 25 percent one-time rise. The 1990 budget summit further increased the deductible to $100 per year, although this level is still below the deductible amounts often associated with private insurance for the under-65 population. The impacts of this and other legislated changes are shown in table 4.1.[1]

For Part A, Hospital Insurance, the deductible rose by about 12 percent beginning in 1982 through a technical change in the formula. Although the hospital deductible increase was proportionally smaller than that for Part B, the dollar amounts were greater. More importantly, this increase was permanently incorporated into the calculation of the deductible, so that its impact rises each year as hospital costs rise. That adjustment thus effectively increased the Part A deductible by $28 in 1982, but by about $78 in 1991 over what it otherwise would have been. The Part A deductible is $736 in 1996, higher than the deductible in most private insurance policies. In addition, since coinsurance for Part A for both hospital and skilled nursing facility (SNF)

Table 4.1 SOURCES OF INCREASED ENROLLEE LIABILITY FOR MEDICARE
          BENEFITS, 1991

	Per Capita Amounts ($)
Total enrollee liability[a]	1,110
Direct increase in liability from changes in:	
Part B premiums	156
Part A deductibles and coinsurance[b]	48
Part B deductible	31
Miscellaneous[c]	−25
Total increase	210
Medicare's net contribution[d]	3,598

Source: Author's estimates extrapolated from Congressional Budget Office and Health Care Financing Administration data.

a. Includes cost sharing, Part B premiums, and excess physician charges.
b. Includes impact of the Prospective Payment System on deductibles, as well as direct increase.
c. Includes radiology/pathology changes, balance billing changes, and others.
d. Net of Part B premium contributions.

care is tied to the deductible, these charges displayed similar proportional increases.

The hospital prospective payment system (PPS) also increased the Part A deductible. Until 1986, the average daily cost of a hospital stay served as the basis for calculating the deductible and coinsurance amounts. But since PPS helped induce shorter lengths of stay, the average cost per hospital day rose faster than before, as more tests and procedures were delivered in a shorter period of time, particularly in the early years of the program. Consequently, the average daily cost rose faster than the overall costs of the program. The deductible amount increased from $400 to $492 between 1985 and 1986—a 23 percent rise in just one year. If, instead, the deductible had risen at the same rate as per capita costs of hospital care over the period, the 1986 deductible would have been only $430.[2] All the coinsurance amounts tied to the Part A deductible would have been smaller as well.

The Omnibus Budget Reconciliation Act of 1986 recognized this problem and changed the deductible formula to reflect increases in costs per case rather than per diem. That change returned the growth in the deductible to a calculation more in tune with the overall cost growth in hospital services. The formula now uses the hospital update factor and case mix index to raise the amount each year. After 1986, rates of growth in the deductible returned to an average annual rate of 5 percent. Nonetheless, the high rates of increase in 1985 and 1986 remain in the base, so that the 1991 deductible of $628 was about $80 above the level it would have been if the 1986 formula had taken effect simultaneously with the advent of PPS.

Together, the two sets of changes affecting the Part A deductible raised the amount paid by beneficiaries by approximately $146 in 1991. Without these two changes, the deductible would have been about $482.

These increases in cost sharing are likely to be covered by the "Medigap" policies that many individuals carry. But that does not mean the burdens are not real to Medicare enrollees, since these higher charges translate directly into premium increases for supplemental policies.[3] Thus, directly or indirectly, most enrollees who use health services were affected by these legislated changes, and their healthcare burdens rose accordingly.

The largest beneficiary cost increase in the 1980s resulted from changes in the formula for calculating the premium for Part B services. When enacted in 1965, beneficiaries were required to pay one-half the costs of Part B insurance coverage. But the rapid increase in the costs of the program outstripped the growth in Social Security benefits. The 1972 Social Security Amendments limited the rate of increase in premiums to the rate of growth in the consumer price index used each year to calculate Social Security cost-of-living increases. Since the cost of Part B services continued to rise at double-digit rates through the end of the 1970s, Part B premiums came to represent a smaller and smaller share of the total costs of the program.

Legislation in 1982 reversed this trend and set the premium at 25 percent of the costs of the program (for elderly beneficiaries) for three years. That requirement has been extended several times; in 1990, the requirement was implicitly renewed through 1995 by setting the specific premium rates for what was then estimated to be 25 percent of the program's costs. By 1991, the premium would have risen to only about $16.90 per month under the 1972 calculations, so the 1991 monthly premium of $29.90 cost beneficiaries about $156 more for the year. That figure has continued to rise each year. In fact, the 1990 legislation overestimated how fast Part B spending would rise, so that by 1995, the premium of $46.10 per month actually represented 31.5 percent of program costs. In 1996, the premium again returned to 25 percent of costs and so for the first time ever, the Part B premium fell, to $42.50.[4]

Offsetting Reductions in Beneficiary Burdens

Other changes in Medicare reduced out-of-pocket burdens on the elderly, but not nearly enough to offset the increases just discussed.[5] Enrollees benefited particularly from federal activities to limit spending for physician services. Both the level of the premiums and the amount of the Part B cost sharing are tied to Medicare spending and hence to allowed charges. So if such charges rise more slowly because of policy, cost sharing will also be limited. For example, the freeze on physician payments for fiscal year 1985 (and extended through May 1986) meant that beneficiaries' cost sharing per visit was also frozen. During 1985, however, per capita expenditures on physician services grew at a rate in excess of 10 percent, suggesting that some physicians may have billed for more complex procedures or may have seen patients more frequently in response to the freeze (Ways and Means 1991). Savings to beneficiaries from this source thus were limited.

Of greater impact were policies designed to restrain beneficiaries' liabilities beyond Medicare's allowed charges. These extra bills accounted for about 16 percent of beneficiary cost sharing in 1985 (Ways and Means 1991). In the mid-1970s, the proportion of bills being accepted on assignment dipped from over 60 percent to about 50 percent and showed little change through the early 1980s. When extra billing did occur, charges usually averaged between 20 percent and 30 percent above Medicare's allowed amounts.[6]

The legislation that established the freeze on physicians' prevailing charges also offered preferential treatment for physicians who agreed to accept Medicare's reasonable-charge determination as full payment for services (i.e., accepted "assignment"). As indicated in the previous chapter, such physicians are termed "participating" physicians if they *always* accept Medicare's allowed charges as payment in full. Although this legislation did not offer full protection from "balance billing," it did help to turn around the trend toward low assignment rates. The result has been a steady increase in the number of physicians who do not charge patients additional fees for their services. HCFA estimated that between 1984 and 1985, excess (or balance) billing for physician claims fell by $16 for the average enrollee—a decline of 16 percent in just one year. By 1991, participating physicians accounted for 73 percent of total Medicare spending, and by January 1, 1992, 52.2 percent of all physicians had signed participation agreements (Physician Payment Review Commission 1992).

Over the next few years, rates of assignment continued to rise, providing an important source of relief to beneficiaries (see figure 4.2). This was one of the few important examples of better protection against the impact of higher costs on Medicare beneficiaries. Participation rates by physicians still vary across both specialties and location, meaning that some beneficiaries may still have difficulty in finding participating physicians. But each year that problem is diminishing. By 1995, 95 percent of all Medicare claims were paid on assignment and 72 percent of providers took part in the participating physician and supplier program (PPRC 1996).

Legislation enacted when the fee freeze was lifted also limited what physicians who chose to continue to balance bill patients could charge. Termed the maximum allowable actual charge (MAAC), the formula was extremely complicated, and its actual impact is thus difficult to assess. But the goal was to place a cap on the amount that physicians could balance bill (Ways and Means 1988). Few physicians and perhaps few carriers understood how the MAAC worked, so it may not have operated as a binding constraint. It has now been replaced by much simpler, and likely more effective, limits—as part of

Figure 4.2 ASSIGNMENT RATES FOR PART B CLAIMS FOR MEDICARE,
            CY 1969–94

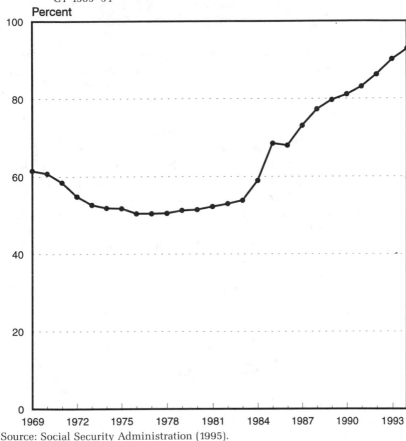

Source: Social Security Administration (1995).

Medicare's physician payment reform. Ultimately, nonparticipating physicians will only be allowed to charge patients 15 percent above their allowed amount—an amount set at 95 percent of that paid to participating physicians.

Overall, balance billing declined as a share of total Medicare costs between 1980 and 1985, and again in 1990 (Ways and Means 1991). The average balance billing amount per beneficiary was $112 per enrollee in 1990, representing almost no real growth since 1985 (during a period of rapid growth in physician spending) (Ways and Means 1991). If the relationship between Part B copayments and balance billing had stayed the same in 1990 as in 1980, the billing limits would have been $148—$36 higher than what occurred. Thus, substantial progress was made in holding down this source of out-of-pocket spending. In 1993, balance billing averaged only $15 per beneficiary (HCFA 1995).

Physician payment reform also resulted in savings to some beneficiaries. Legislative changes in 1987 and 1989 previewed the reforms with cuts in "overvalued" procedures. These changes brought about some of the reductions at the high end, but without raising the "undervalued" procedures. These changes led to substantial reductions in the fees for affected procedures (Zuckerman and Holahan 1992). For example, although most prices for physician services increase each year, sonography and ambulatory eye procedures each declined by over 3 percent between 1987 and 1988, when substantial shares of those procedures were subject to the policy changes.

The Medicare physician payment reform legislation, on the other hand, was intended to be "budget neutral" in terms of physician reimbursement, meaning that the increases in fees established for some physicians are offset by decreases for others. Consequently, the impact across all beneficiaries should also be budget neutral for the basic fee schedule, although there will be individual gainers and losers. Those gaining the most are beneficiaries undergoing surgical and other procedures where payments are being substantially cut. The big losers are individuals with chronic illnesses who are heavy users of physician office visits, since each dollar of increase in physician charges for an office visit translates into a 20-cent increase in required cost sharing. In simulating the impact of these changes, Mitchell and Menke (1990) found little variation across definable population groups. About the only noticeable change was for rural residents who would, on average, "lose" under the fee schedule. On the other hand, the balance billing limits that were also part of the legislation have resulted in savings for beneficiaries that are enough to offset most losses from higher fees.[7] The biggest gainers from the physician payment limits according to Mitchell and Menke's simulations would be beneficiaries who are hospitalized, largely because balance billing (the discrepancy between the Medicare allowed charge and prevailing charges) tends to be higher than average among specialists and surgeons.

The increase in the numbers of participating physicians and the lower balance billing does not mean, however, that all physicians have been happy with the controls they face over what they can bill patients. Indeed, the 1995 Balanced Budget Act (which was vetoed by President Clinton) contained provisions that physicians lobbied strongly for to soften restrictions on balance billing. This issue may well emerge again in future reforms of Medicare.

DISTRIBUTION OF THE IMPACT

The combined impact of these benefit and cost-sharing changes led to a reduction in Medicare benefits of about 5 percent in 1991— compared to what would have occurred if no changes had been made in Medicare policy—and a 19 percent increase in enrollee liability for Medicare-covered services.[8] The shift in liability from Medicare to its enrollees as a result of the policy changes discussed above averaged about $210 in 1991 (see table 4.1).

But not all Medicare enrollees were affected equally. Needs and use of care vary dramatically across individuals; so, too, do the resulting financial burdens. For example, a Medicare beneficiary with an extended hospital stay would pay nearly $400 more in a given year as a result of these changes.

One way to systematically look at some of this variation is to consider age differences. The heaviest users of healthcare services are the oldest beneficiaries—the group that is also rising the fastest within the Medicare population (see table 4.2). They are particularly heavy users of Part A services, with skilled nursing care leading the list. Persons aged 85 and above are over 800 percent more likely to use Medicare skilled nursing facility (SNF) benefits than those aged 65 to 74. Next in importance for the "oldest old" is home health.

Table 4.2 USE OF MEDICARE SERVICES FOR 1,000 MEDICARE ENROLLEES, BY AGE: 1993

Age of Enrollee	Ratio Compared to Age 65–74 Group			
	Hospital Inpatient: Discharges	Skilled Nursing Services: Covered Admissions	Home Health: Persons Served	Physician Services: Users
65–74	1.00	1.00	1.00	1.00
75–84	1.54	3.52	2.44	1.17
85 and above	1.98	8.38	4.09	1.28
Disabled	1.50	0.88	1.08	0.95

Source: HCFA (1995).

Use of physician services (Part B) is considerably less correlated with age. Persons over age 85 are only 28 percent more likely to see a physician than is a beneficiary between the ages of 65 and 74 (see table 4.2). This is an especially dramatic statistic, given the higher use of hospital care by older beneficiaries, suggesting that ambulatory visits are much less important for older than for younger beneficiaries.

Dollar expenditures display a similar pattern. The oldest beneficiaries always have higher expenditures than younger ones (table 4.3). The differences are greatest for Part A services, with skilled nursing and home health benefits most often used by those who have complications—including frailty associated with age—that lengthens periods of recovery from acute illnesses. Disabled beneficiaries have expenditures more like those aged 75 to 84 than like younger nondisabled beneficiary groups.

Thus, only premium changes are age neutral, that is, affecting all beneficiaries equally. Any change in cost-sharing or reimbursement policy that affects beneficiaries in one part of the program and not another will have differential effects by age. Changes in physician cost sharing will be more evenly distributed by age and will vary less within each age group than changes in coinsurance, since most Medicare beneficiaries (about 80 percent) have reimbursable Medicare physician expenses. This is particularly true for changes in the Part B deductible, as opposed to the coinsurance, which will fall more heavily on those with heavy use. (And since heavy users of physician services are also very likely to have a hospital stay, they will suffer the double burden of having cost-sharing liability from both parts of the program.)

What about the specific burdens of the direct changes in beneficiary cost sharing implemented during the 1980s? About three-quarters of the direct changes described in table 4.1 were spread evenly across most enrollees. These include the changes in the Part B premium and

Table 4.3 VARIATIONS IN MEDICARE OUT-OF-POCKET LIABILITIES, BY AGE, 1993

Age of Enrollee	Average Liability	Ratio to Age 65–74
Disabled	$1,151	1.24
65–74	926	1.00
75–84	1,151	1.24
85 and above	1,312	1.42
All Enrollees	1,055	—

Source: HCFA (1995).

the Part B deductible. The Part A deductible and coinsurance increases and the change in radiology and pathology services (felt by those who are hospitalized) fell disproportionately on older beneficiaries, who are also those least able to afford the higher burdens of cost sharing.

At the end of the 1980s, a new program, the Qualified Medicare Beneficiary benefit, was added as part of the 1988 Catastrophic legislation (the subject of the next chapter). This benefit, which survived the repeal of that legislation, is actually part of the Medicaid program but was designed to specifically aid low-income and asset beneficiaries who are Medicare eligible with the costs of cost sharing and Part B premiums. This program has helped to ease some of the financial burdens on elderly and disabled persons, although the rate of participation among eligibles is rather low. For example, 4 to 5 percent of elderly and disabled persons who otherwise would not receive Medicaid protection are aided by this program, which provides relief for the $1,261 average Medicare liabilities that beneficiaries faced in 1995.

PPS AND INDIRECT BURDENS ON BENEFICIARIES

Overall, savings to the federal budget from Medicare changes directed at providers have been about twice the level of savings from changes that have fallen directly on beneficiaries. For instance, in the changes from the 1990 budget summit, the balance of provider-to-beneficiary changes (Ways and Means 1990) was 3 to 1. Nonetheless, the implicit consequences of some of the changes targeted to providers increase costs to beneficiaries as well.

The most significant single provider change implemented in the 1980s was the introduction of the hospital Prospective Payment System (PPS). This serves as a compelling case study for the relevance of examining beneficiary impacts. In many respects, the introduction of PPS has likely brought about more efficient delivery of care with no adverse consequences on beneficiaries. For example, prior to PPS, the old cost-based reimbursement system was widely criticized as promoting lengthy hospital stays for Medicare patients. Stays would sometimes even be extended for patients' (or relatives') convenience rather than for sound medical reasons. Eliminating these extra days would improve efficiency, lower costs, and actually prove beneficial to patients if earlier discharge reduced their risk of developing hospital-based infections. But other PPS-induced changes may have merely shifted the costs of care onto the beneficiaries or reduced the quality of service, as hospitals changed their behavior in response to PPS. The true efficiency effects of the reduced costs of providing healthcare should be distinguished from those that sacrifice quality or merely shift burdens.

To develop specific estimates of the impacts of such changes on beneficiaries constitutes a formidable task. Causation is difficult to establish, and some of the "costs" are intangible (as noted) and thus hard to measure. Yet such efforts are needed to fully evaluate the impact of provider changes.

The three major sources of potential burdens to beneficiaries from PPS—shorter hospital stays, shifting the site of service, and less care while in the hospital—are discussed here in turn.

Effects of Shorter Hospital Stays

Perhaps most important of all these changes has been the movement toward shorter hospital stays by Medicare patients. Hospitals are paid the same amount for a particular type of admission (by diagnosis-related group [DRG]), whether the patient stays 5 or 10 days, for example. And the length of the hospital stay is one of the simplest elements for a hospital to control. Further, the trend in length of stay (LOS) had been downward for some time, for Medicare beneficiaries as well as the population in general. The response to PPS was a substantial acceleration of that trend, as shown in figure 4.3. From 1983 to 1985, average hospital stays for Medicare patients fell from 9.7 to 8.7 days, a decline of over 10 percent (NCHS 1991).

The quality issue raised by these shorter lengths of stay is whether they represent desirable or undesirable changes in medical practice. Changes in medical practice and in procedures themselves led to at least some of the historical decline in LOS. New techniques often speed recovery and reduce the need for long hospital stays. Moreover, hospitals are dangerous places where risks of postoperative infection may be high; in general, patients recover better at home. On the other hand, when patients are told that their DRGs "have run out," the discharges may reflect hospitals' budgetary concerns more than patient needs. Although hospitals are supposed to keep patients as long as medically necessary, and there is technically no such thing as DRGs "running out" for patients, hospitals make such claims to hold the line on costs. If patients are discharged too early, they face higher risks of dying, of being readmitted to the hospital, or of taking longer to recover at home, the "quicker and sicker" issue. In addition, as

Figure 4.3 AVERAGE LENGTH OF STAY IN NONFEDERAL SHORT-STAY
HOSPITALS, BY AGE, 1980–93

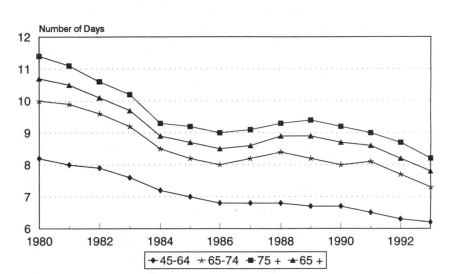

Source: NCHS (1995, 1991).

noted, they may need follow-up services to substitute for hospital care—services not covered as part of this policy change.

Thus far, only a few studies have examined the impact of PPS, and then only for the early years of the program. What is more, most studies have looked at only the crudest indicators of quality—mortality rates and rates of readmission. A worsening of these statistics would suggest severe problems from PPS. Studies of mortality have failed to detect any significant changes (Coulam and Gaumer 1991).

The most dramatic findings on PPS's impact on readmissions come from a study by the RAND Corporation (Kahn et al. 1990).[9] Despite a relatively positive overall assessment of PPS, the results were mixed. The RAND study found that for four of the health conditions studied, readmissions fell post-PPS, while increasing for myocardial infarction (Kahn et al. 1990). The study also found that patients were discharged earlier and sicker after the introduction of PPS. There was a 22 percent increase in the proportion of beneficiaries discharged in an unstable condition after PPS, compared to a similar pre-PPS group (Kosekoff et al. 1990).[10] And for those discharged home, instead of to an institutional setting, there was a 43 percent increase in instability. These findings portend undesirable health outcomes as well, since the study also found that instability at discharge was associated with a higher probability of dying within 30 days.[11]

What about greater reliance on other less-intensive care? Shifting the type of service is not necessarily an undesirable outcome, if such services are available. But no specific provisions were made to enhance the availability of such care after the introduction of PPS, so beneficiaries had to rely on the existing supply of services. Both SNF and home health under Medicare were tightly controlled in the mid-1980s by conservative interpretations of regulations. In addition, the tightened requirements for reimbursement made some nursing homes and home health agencies reluctant to take on some patients, for fear of being denied reimbursement. To the extent that this represented a major constraint, PPS may have caused early discharges in which patients lacked access to needed "step-down" care. Alternatively, some patients may have received care but crowded out other traditional recipients of nursing home or community-based services (Wood and Estes 1990).

In 1985, there were 22.8 million fewer hospital days as compared to 1983. On average, about one-third of this decrease affected Medicare beneficiaries with long-term care needs who were likely to require further assistance in recuperating from a hospital stay.[12] But the number of Medicare-funded SNF visits actually decreased from 1984 to 1988 in response to restrictive Medicare coverage provisions implemented in 1984 (Feinglass and Holloway 1991). In fact, in 1987 covered days of care for SNFs were only 81 percent of the 1983 level, despite growth in the number of Medicare beneficiaries. Converting this figure to days per 1,000 elderly beneficiaries indicates that coverage declined from 338 to 248 over the period, meaning that benefits per enrollee in 1987 were only 73.4 percent of the 1983 level (Silverman 1991).

Home health visits increased over this period. But the *rate* of growth in these visits declined after PPS (Kenney 1991). PPS stimulated use of home health over what it would have been otherwise, but from a declining base. Home health visits per 1,000 enrollees also declined by 7.4 percent between 1983 and 1988. Although SNF and home health constituted only a small piece of Part A in the mid- to late 1980s, the demands generated by PPS for follow-up care should have increased use of SNF and home health services after 1983. Instead, increases in spending for these two services were at or below their pre-PPS average rates of change between 1983 and 1985.

Together, Medicare SNF and home health benefits did not rise enough to replace the number of hospital days lost under PPS. To the extent that individuals obtained noncovered services such as home-maker services or did without needed services, beneficiary burdens increased accordingly through the "quicker and sicker" side effects of PPS. Studies do not find dramatic impacts on mortality, but there are indications that early discharge may create problems, particularly related to quality of life.

Shifting the Site of Service

Inpatient admission rates for Medicare enrollees fell dramatically after the introduction of PPS and continued to fall throughout the 1980s. Some procedures that used to be performed on an inpatient basis, such as cataract surgery, are now done almost exclusively in outpatient settings, a change that would likely have occurred without PPS, albeit perhaps more slowly. Between 1980 and 1989, the number of inpatient surgeries for extraction of a lens decreased from 335,000 to 60,000 (NCHS 1991). But on the outpatient side, that same procedure increased even more. Expenditures on ambulatory eye procedures, dominated by cataract surgery, grew at an annual rate of 13.3 percent from 1985 to 1989, much of that accounted for by increased volume and intensity (Zuckerman and Holahan 1992).

Shifting surgery and other major procedures to the outpatient setting reflects, to some degree, changes in these procedures that make them safer and easier. For example, laser surgery of the eye has led to remarkable improvements in cataract surgery. Thus it is not surprising that these are now almost universally outpatient procedures. But very frail patients or those with poor home circumstances that may impede recovery may be placed at a disadvantage when operations are performed only in outpatient settings. The shift outside of the hospital seems to have occurred with equal frequency for beneficiaries of all ages, suggesting that treating different patient characteristics differently has not played a major role in the decision making (Leader and Moon 1989).

Effects of Less Inpatient Care

Enrollees will not receive needed care if, in response to PPS, hospitals become reluctant to accept some types of patients and physicians do not press for these admissions. In some cases, people who were previously hospitalized for tests or treatment are now getting less care or care of a different sort. Although there has been an increase in the severity of the condition of patients treated in the hospital setting since the introduction of PPS, use of technology has remained largely unchanged (Sloan, Morrisey, and Valvona 1988).[13] Chesney (1990) found that the composition of patients using intensive care units (ICUs) did not change after the introduction of PPS, but that the severity of patients *not* admitted to ICUs did increase. What is not clear is whether less care received during the stay resulted in adverse outcomes. These reductions may reflect more efficient care—a desired result of PPS.

These analyses suggest that PPS did shift provider incentives to a preference for less, rather than more, care. Fewer resources are now directed to patients (at a given severity level) in terms of length of stay, technologies used, and even decisions to admit to the hospital. Interestingly, many of these trends have carried over to non-Medicare patients as well. Often these reductions may actually be desirable. And even when they are not, the problems may be related more to a lack of step-down care than to PPS itself. In the past, errors were made on the side of delivering too much care. Now the incentive is to provide too little. Such changes are inevitable in an environment of concern about controlling costs, but they also raise the need for heightened oversight of quality.

QUALITY OF CARE

In the early days of Medicare, little emphasis was placed on quality of care. If access to mainstream care were assured, it was reasoned, Medicare enrollees would enjoy the best in healthcare that the nation could offer, and quality would be a "nonissue." Spurred in part by a changing climate for healthcare in general and Medicare in particular, interest in quality issues has been on the increase. Part of the concern arose with introduction of PPS—it was felt that more vigilance was required when there were incentives to use less care in hospital settings. Beyond the effect of PPS, there has been some scrutiny of the impact of the new Medicare Fee Schedule on physician payment and enrollees' participation in health maintenance organizations (HMOs). Another source of concern for quality has arisen from questions about cost-effectiveness in general. Is some care not only unnecessary but harmful? At least in this instance, quality improvements and cost containment would be compatible. Finally, some health researchers have raised alarms about the lack of self-enforcement of standards by providers, allowing problems to go undetected and/or uncorrected.

Medicare Physician Payment Reform and Quality

A major issue for the quality of care in the early 1990s centered on the question of whether physician payment reform would reduce beneficiaries' access to care. Concern was expressed that doctors who faced lower fees might respond by having patients return more frequently for visits and procedures, by spending less time with patients on any given visit, or by refusing to take Medicare patients. The assumptions that led the Health Care Financing Administration (HCFA) to project a "behavioral response" to the Fee Schedule implied that physicians would increase the volume of their businesses, charging for more visits and procedures. That would likely mean less time on each activity and perhaps subjecting patients to unnecessary and sometimes risky procedures. And initially there seemed to be anecdotal evidence suggesting that lowered fees would cause doctors to substitute other patients and refuse to take on new Medicare patients—or perhaps even turn away existing Medicare patients (Freudenheim 1992). This was a particular concern in underserved areas where patients have little choice in what doctor to see. Further reduction of access to care in such areas could exacerbate some of the regional variations in use of services.

In an attempt to determine whether beneficiaries have problems in access to care as a result of the Medicare Fee Schedule, the HCFA has been interviewing beneficiaries each year. Between 1991 and 1993, beneficiaries reported a decrease in barriers to access and an increase in overall satisfaction with the Medicare program (Rosenbach et al. 1995). The survey found beneficiaries reporting greater ease in getting to a doctor, with only about 7 percent of beneficiaries having a problem. Moreover, patients of all types reported relatively consistent abilities to access care, with some of the discrepancies by race and income diminishing over time. The greatest improvement in access occurred in reports about satisfaction concerning the cost of physician services.

Access still remains an issue in a few geographic areas, however. For example, in northwest Arizona; Boise, Idaho; and Fort Worth, Texas (PPRC 1996). But these areas show access to be a problem for all persons in a given area, suggesting that the problem is physician supply rather than discrimination against Medicare patients.

HMOs and Quality

In the 1980s, the Medicare program embraced the prospect of achieving cost savings through enrollee participation in health maintenance organizations, first as an experiment and then as a permanent part of the program. Qualified HMOs that choose to participate must take any Medicare enrollee who applies. They must cover at least the same benefits as Medicare. As described in chapter 3, enrollment in these plans has begun to accelerate in the 1990s.

There are many potential advantages to enrollment in HMOs. As inducements, beneficiaries often receive broader coverage than Medicare offers. HMO plans sometimes require no additional premiums (beyond the standard Part B premium) and at most, charge amounts less than comparable Medigap plans. Filing of claims is eliminated, and cost sharing is usually reduced and simplified.[14] Moreover, a high-quality HMO can provide good coordination of care and help to patients in wending their way through the healthcare system.

On the other hand, just as PPS raised issues of quality in a system that offers incentives to reduce the level of care offered, HMOs and other capitated systems pose similar concerns. Since Medicare essentially turns over all responsibility to the HMO, it does not receive any information of the quantity of care received and thus cannot track whether appropriate services are being delivered. In addition, the process of developing standards for evaluating HMOs has been painfully slow.

The Health Care Financing Administration is in the process of working with the private sector to refine measures for assessing the quality of care in HMOs, but no results are expected for some time. In 1996, HCFA plans to disseminate information comparing premiums and benefits in these plans—basic information that is not now routinely available. There has also been very little work on identifying other problems and unresolved issues arising under Medicare HMOs, although anecdotal evidence abounds. One key is the extent to which beneficiaries choose to disenroll from an HMO when there is a problem. Since this is possible on a nearly continuous basis, disenrollment may be an indicator of potential problems. A recent study of those who disenrolled found some problems with HMOs, but a reasonable level of overall performance (Inspector General 1995).

There have been some notable failures in the Medicare HMO program, particularly in the early years of the program when, to encourage HMOs to participate, exceptions were granted to established standards. Several dramatic failures in the late 1980s, such as that of IMC in Florida, cast doubt on HCFA's oversight (U.S. General Accounting Office 1992).

The track record for the industry has since improved, however, and well-established HMOs have been able to effectively serve beneficiaries. While the proportion of beneficiaries enrolled in HMOs—just over 10 percent—remains small, rapid growth in participation makes the issue of developing strong quality assessment tools and providing that information to beneficiaries particularly important. At present, beneficiaries do not even receive notices about the availability of plans, and Medicare has no information to aid those who wish to choose an HMO option. In this regard, Medicare lags behind the private sector.

Peer Review Organizations

Medicare established Peer Review Organizations (PROs) for two reasons: to oversee use of services for purposes of cost containment and to monitor the quality of care received by Medicare beneficiaries.[15] By most accounts, PROs have concentrated on this first mission, often to the detriment of the quality-control portion. PRO contracts with HCFA have generally specified that much of their time be spent on activities such as hospital preadmission screening, sampling of inpatient records, and DRG validation. Although these activities may have quality components, the emphasis certainly has been more on controlling the use of services. In addition, PRO activities have focused primarily on hospitals; there is almost no oversight of ambulatory services.

Current PRO procedures have come in for considerable criticism as quality oversight mechanisms. Use of generic screens tends to result in review of many cases, bogging down the process in paperwork. Moreover, at the end of the process, PROs have little flexibility in the types of sanctions they can use against offending physicians or institutions; the choice is between severe sanctions or none at all. Moreover, all of the PROs' monitoring activities focus on care received. To the extent that problems also arise from lack of care, Medicare has no tracking mechanisms or ability to oversee problems. Thus, much of the quality effort is directly tied to what is done for Medicare enrollees, and hence is linked to some notion of effectiveness. PROs look for errors of commission, but not errors of omission. No broader assessments are made regarding what the level of overall care should be. For example, in evaluating the PPS, there is no mechanism for assessing whether too little care is being delivered or whether some who should be admitted to hospitals have been excluded.

The PRO program could be substantially improved to better serve the Medicare enrollee population. A 1990 report by the Institute of Medicine detailed recommendations to shift the focus of quality assessment and assurance by Medicare away from the current punitive, adversarial approach that focuses on outliers rather than the overall standard of care (Lohr 1990). The report advocated a new system that would enlarge the role of Medicare in quality, in part by expanding the definition of quality of care, by redirecting the activities of the PROs, by emphasizing improved research and measurement of quality issues, and by preparing professionals to address such issues. A gradual process was stressed, using the existing PRO structure. In many cases, the recommendations were not specific, since many of the ideas for improving quality were as yet untested. Furthermore, considerable federal investment of funds would be required.

No formal efforts have yet been undertaken to institute these changes or to otherwise expand the PRO system. Implementation of HCFA's goal to expand PRO activities to assess quality in ambulatory settings or in HMOs has also been slow in coming. Some areas of improvement that were stressed by the Institute of Medicine's report are now underway, however. In particular, analysis of the effectiveness of medical care is now a recognized goal of the government health research community.

Using Effectiveness Studies to Improve Quality

In the late 1980s the promise of achieving cost savings while also enhancing quality came to be associated with research on the effectiveness or appropriateness of healthcare. For example, an early study by the RAND Corporation on carotid endarterectomies suggested that this procedure was often inappropriately performed, not only raising Medicare costs but also potentially harming patients who were exposed to unnecessary risks from this major surgical procedure (Merrick et al. 1986). Later studies of coronary artery bypass (Winslow et al. 1988) and coronary angiography (Chassin et al. 1987) came to similar conclusions. The suggestion that there is not only a considerable amount of unnecessary surgery, but that it could be identified and its prevalence reduced, was welcome news to many seeking "magic bullets" to achieve healthcare savings. Indeed, some researchers have argued that healthcare costs could be reduced by as much as

20 percent or 30 percent if such unnecessary procedures could be eliminated.

One tangible indicator of the enthusiasm of the policy world for such solutions was the dramatic increase in funding for effectiveness research by the federal government. Millions of dollars of new monies were targeted for these studies, and the National Center for Health Services Research changed its name to the Agency for Health Care Policy and Research (AHCPR) and reoriented its research agenda to focus support on this effort.

One caution was sounded, however, by a pioneer in this research, Robert Brook, who argued that although overuse of services is a problem in some areas, further study would also identify areas of underuse that suggest we should spend more and not less to achieve high-quality care (Brook et al. 1989).

There will likely be a long lag before findings on research effectiveness are available and disseminated widely enough to have any noticeable impact on behavior. That is not to say that there will not be impacts eventually. The case of Cesarean sections for childbirth indicates the promise. Dissemination of information about the excessive reliance on that procedure has indeed had an impact on the proportion of births delivered by Cesarean section in recent years, although it took a combination of empirical evidence and efforts to publicize the results to change behavior (Myers and Gleicher 1988).

Most of the research of AHCPR has thus far focused on the development of practice guidelines for specific problems. Funding was greatly expanded in the first half of the 1990s. But controversy over some of the results and general skepticism about government research has recently prompted a less favorable view of the agency, putting the future role of public support for such research in doubt.

Program Satisfaction

Quality of care under Medicare can be broadly defined to encompass many concerns. One concern yet to be discussed relates to beneficiary satisfaction. How well does Medicare meet perceived needs? Can "user-friendly" improvements help boost the perceived quality of the program? And what about broader concerns relating to coverage of services under Medicare?

Medicare fares relatively well in measures of consumer satisfaction. Polls generally indicate that the program is popular with beneficiaries and that they are happy with their doctors and the care they receive. Their major complaints often center on the program's unclear explanation of benefits and communication problems in seeking information regarding when services are to be covered and in lodging complaints. These are certainly less critical issues than standard quality concerns, but they ought to be addressed by the program. Cost sharing makes considerable paperwork almost inevitable, but simplification and clarification of forms could aid beneficiaries. Funding for administration under Medicare has also been constrained in this period of cost containment; such constraints seem likely to continue. Nevertheless, minimal expenditures in this area could pay considerable dividends in patient satisfaction. For example, more rapid response to queries or complaints and improved forms might reduce the time burdens on individuals in dealing with the system without causing substantial extra outlays on administration.

The other major source of dissatisfaction with Medicare—its lack of coverage for specific kinds of care—would be much more expensive to resolve. By excluding certain key types of healthcare services, enrollees may not get a well-rounded course of treatment or may misuse the system to make up for its shortcomings. For example, exclusion of prescription drug coverage under Medicare may result in patients who have access to physicians but are unable to comply with a course of treatment if they cannot afford the increasingly expensive drugs that the doctor prescribes. Although drugs may often be an extremely cost-effective way to treat certain conditions, this is one area where patients with limited means skimp on care. The result may be unnecessarily more intensive care later when the problem is left untreated. Is this a Medicare quality problem? For many beneficiaries, the answer is yes.

Lack of coverage of long-term and chronic care is particularly likely to lead to poor quality outcomes. Lack of coverage for supportive services may result in more hospitalization and treatment in the acute-care setting than would occur if coverage were not an issue. Before PPS, long hospital stays may have been, in part, a reflection of lack of options for follow-up care by Medicare enrollees. Inappropriate use of services can be harmful—for example, patients may be exposed to greater risk of infection as inpatients, while still not getting care that is most relevant to their needs. On the other hand, the fact that such patients are now discharged earlier may simply mean that they return home with inadequate support, also an undesirable outcome.

The lack of coverage of important services raises troubling problems in assessing the quality of care under Medicare. How do we separate outcomes that are due to poor quality of Medicare services from problems that may arise because of the services excluded from Medicare?

For example, if a beneficiary does not receive appropriate drugs because Medicare does not offer prescription drug coverage and the person cannot afford to pay for the drugs, adverse outcomes such as avoidable hospitalization may occur. While Medicare may be doing a good job within the limits of the services that it offers, an outcomes-based standard for quality of care would not make this distinction.

CONCLUSIONS

Although, ironically, Medicare is one of the most popular of all government programs, it has also been subject to large and continuing budget cuts. How can we reconcile these two facts? Many analysts argue that since cuts in the program have largely been directed at providers, beneficiaries have not been affected. However, this overstates the degree to which beneficiaries have been insulated from change.

Medicare cost sharing liability for enrollees has risen substantially compared to its level in 1980. Some of this has resulted from direct increases in premiums, deductibles, and coinsurance, the cumulative and continuing effects of which reduce Medicare payments significantly.

As Medicare clamps down on providers and experiments with new ways to hold down costs, it is likely to influence the quality of care received as well. For example, earlier hospital discharges may place the frail and vulnerable elderly at greater risk of death or complications, suggesting that enrollees have an important stake in the broad range of cost-containment strategies pursued by the government. The physician payment fee schedule may also affect access to certain services—especially if payment levels are further restricted. And HMOs remain a black box with little information available on quality.

Fortunately, Medicare in the early 1980s started from a base of high-quality care, with generous payments to providers and a substantial subsidy provided to enrollees. Thus, erosions in financial support or in the quality of care need to be assessed against this initial base. Nonetheless, it is incorrect to argue that Medicare cuts have been painless for enrollees. Nor are beneficiaries likely to be satisfied simply with the knowledge that erosion in quality has been small.

Most of these changes have failed to ignite the passions of elderly and disabled persons. One change did—the Medicare Catastrophic Coverage Act (MCCA) of 1988, which was designed to expand Medicare's reach.[16] A new era in Medicare policy began with the passage and nearly instant revocation of the MCCA. The controversy over the MCCA—and its pivotal implications for future Medicare policy—are the subject of the next chapter.

Notes

1. Assessing the cumulative effects of these many changes is a difficult task. Savings in each year reflect assumptions about the growth in benefits over time that are not constant. Thus, it is difficult, for example, to compare 1982 changes with those made in 1989 and group them all in a table for 1991.

A number of other smaller changes also boosted the proportion of Medicare expenditures that beneficiaries must pay. For instance, hospital-based radiologists' and pathologists' charges used to be fully covered by Medicare. Now, these physicians' fees are subject to the normal 20 percent coinsurance that beneficiaries must pay. In another example, before 1981 some costs of physicians' services from the previous year could be carried over and applied to the current year's deductible. This is no longer allowed.

2. If the increase had been to only $430 in 1986, the effect of the legislation increasing the deductible by 12 percent would have meant a $46 impact. Thus, the indirect impact of PPS on the deductible in 1986 was 35 percent greater than the impact of a change specifically designed to raise the Part A deductible.

3. Some Medicare enrollees have either Medicaid or employer-provided insurance that may render them largely immune to these changes. However, unless the employer fully absorbs the premium costs of the insurance, beneficiaries will bear some of the burden. Most employer-provided coverage requires at least some contribution from the retiree.

4. Legislation in 1993 extended the 25 percent requirement through 1998 when it presumably will again revert to growing at the same rate as the CPI. Legislative proposals in 1995 would have frozen it at 31.5 percent indefinitely, but this was part of the Balanced Budget Act vetoed by President Clinton.

5. Minor changes include the extension of Medicare coverage to include hospice benefits for the terminally ill. Although this broadened the range of choices open to beneficiaries, it represented a very limited expansion. Similarly, as part of a move to establish a fee schedule for independent laboratory services, patient cost sharing was eliminated on July 1, 1984.

6. These additional charges may not always be assessed against the beneficiary. They are the amounts reported to the Health Care Financing Administration; patients may or may not pay all these charges.

7. Mitchell and Menke's (1990) simulations were based on 1986 data, however, when balance billing was relatively more important than it was in 1991, the year before the fee schedule was set to begin. Thus, these results are likely to be more dramatic than what Medicare beneficiaries will experience over the next few years.

8. Although beneficiaries' overall share of Medicare costs actually stayed about the same through the 1980s, that share would otherwise have declined over time if no legislative changes had occurred. This is because the Part B premium was tied to the rate of increase in the Social Security cost-of-living adjustment from 1973 to 1981, which grew more slowly than the costs of Medicare.

9. This effort assessed health outcomes from PPS by contrasting data on 16,758 Medicare patients hospitalized prior to and subsequent to the introduction of PPS in five states. The first set of results focused on five disease categories: congestive heart failure, acute myocardial infarction, pneumonia, cerebrovascular accident, and hip fracture during the first several years of PPS (Kahn et al. 1990).

10. That is, after PPS, 18 percent were discharged in unstable condition, as compared to 15 percent before PPS.

11. Most other studies of such outcomes have been done on a smaller scale and offer a mixed picture. See, for example, Fitzgerald et al. 1987, Palmer et al. 1989, and Gerety, Doderholm-Difatte, and Winograd (1989).

12. This reflects the numbers of Medicare beneficiaries who have chronic health limitations that might normally require special assistance. Early discharges for such individuals would likely require extraordinary help. And, of course, others who have no additional complications might also need assistance if the discharge is truly premature.

13. That is, as easier cases are being treated outside the hospital, the more severe cases are left to the inpatient setting.

14. Although Medicare beneficiaries do not have to file claims for the basic program, they generally do in order to receive reimbursement under their supplemental policies.

15. Effectively, PROs replaced the Professional Standards Review Organizations (PSROs), which were instituted by the 1972 Social Security Amendments. These organizations did some early work on quality-of-care issues, such as auditing medical records to analyze quality problems.

16. Moreover, strong objections to the first package of Medicare cuts in the 1990 budget summit helped send the negotiators back to the drawing board. The final package of Medicare cuts was much less stringent on beneficiaries.

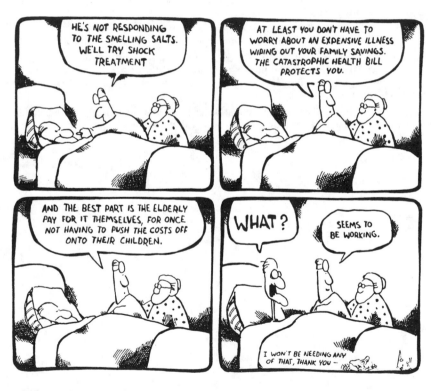

Chapter Five

THE MEDICARE CATASTROPHIC
COVERAGE ACT

The Medicare Catastrophic Coverage Act (MCCA) represents one of the shortest-lived pieces of social legislation in the United States. It also marked a turning point in Medicare policy. Unlike earlier additions to the Medicare legislation, such as the 1972 amendments that added disabled and end-stage renal patients, the Catastrophic Coverage Act was intended to be budget neutral, requiring beneficiaries themselves to fund the additions to benefits. It also constituted a marked departure from earlier proposed legislation of the Reagan years that sought to restrict Medicare coverage and reduce costs at the expense of both providers and beneficiaries. After years of cost-cutting efforts, the MCCA sought to expand Medicare benefits. It also embodied many of the constraints faced by legislation in the 1980s that sought to expand the role of government despite the high federal deficit and the Gramm-Rudman-Hollings budget restrictions. Thus, it must be viewed in a broader political context as well.[1]

The MCCA offers important political and economic lessons. In political terms, the act launched an unprecedented debate about the future of Medicare—as well as of other domestic policy initiatives—that will likely shape policy choices to come. Economically, it became clear that even minor changes in Medicare come with large price tags, and that beneficiaries may well not find the cost worth the benefits as they perceive them, if they are asked to pay a considerable amount of the cost. Further, if new benefits are to be funded by a flat per beneficiary premium (rather than contributions graduated by income) it is impossible to provide benefits generous enough to be of much help. Progressive financing of new Medicare benefits becomes ever more of an issue as elderly beneficiaries become increasingly unequal in their ability to pay for healthcare and other needs.

RECOGNIZING THE NEED FOR CATASTROPHIC PROTECTION

Rapidly rising healthcare costs both generated interest in cost-containment efforts under Medicare and exerted further pressure on elderly and disabled beneficiaries to share more of the costs of their own care. By 1987, cost sharing had increased to the point where elderly beneficiaries were spending about the same share of their incomes on healthcare as they did before Medicare was introduced. A considerable portion of that burden came from the rising deductible and coinsurance requirements of Medicare, as well as the increasing fees for critical services that Medicare did not cover. In 1987, when the MCCA was first being debated, persons aged 65 and over had average per capita expenditures of $5,360 on healthcare, only $3,356 of which came from public sources (i.e., Medicare and Medicaid) (Waldo et al. 1989), implying average out-of-pocket or premium expenses of just over $2,000. The elderly were even liable for nearly a quarter of the costs of hospital and physician services ($726 in 1987), which are relatively well covered by Medicare. They also lacked coverage for nursing home care—the largest source of uncovered services for older persons—and for other crucial healthcare expenditures such as prescription drugs, dental and vision care, and homemaker services. After excluding Medicare out-of-pocket liabilities for covered services, older persons faced an average liability of $1,278 for these other expenditures.

These averages do not capture how high the liabilities can be for persons with even relatively modest health problems. For example, individuals who trigger hospital coinsurance had average out-of-pocket spending for Medicare-covered cost sharing of $7,852 in 1988 (Congressional Budget Office 1987). Beneficiaries who did not trigger the coinsurance but had at least two hospital stays averaged $2,387 in cost-sharing liabilities, not counting spending on other healthcare services that Medicare does not cover.

Many Medicare beneficiaries rely on private supplemental insurance (Medigap) to fill in at least some of these gaps. Insurance companies such as Blue Cross/Blue Shield or organizations such as the American Association of Retired Persons (AARP) offer Medigap policies. Standard plans usually cover the deductibles and coinsurance that Medicare requires, and sometimes small amounts of additional benefits, but the comprehensiveness of the benefit package varies substantially across policies. For example, at considerably higher premiums, drug coverage is sometimes available to individuals. The costs of such additions are high, not only because the benefits are costly, but also because individuals who choose higher coverage are more likely to use the services.

Some fortunate beneficiaries receive coverage as part of retirement benefits. These policies are often either free to the retiree or at least partially subsidized. Benefits are usually more generous under these plans, which are intended to raise coverage to the level held by these individuals when they were active employees. For example, many employer-based plans include prescription drugs. In 1987, about 31 percent of the elderly had such employer-based coverage (NCHSR 1989).

But those most in need of protection—low-income elderly and disabled persons—are the ones least likely to have private supplemental protection. Such individuals tend not to have employer-based coverage and often cannot afford Medigap policies. Given the costs of Medigap, it is surprising that any low-income individuals actually purchase such policies. Moreover, although Medigap has helped smooth out the variations in acute-care liability for those who have it, individuals with coverage spend an even higher share of their incomes on health than if they had no Medigap protection, since they pay high administrative costs for relatively modest protection (Feder et al. 1987a). And for the low-income beneficiaries, comprehensive protection is simply unaffordable. Over half of the elderly (56.2 percent) with incomes of $10,000 or less had out-of-pocket spending totaling more than 15 percent of their incomes in 1986 (Feder et al. 1987b) (see table 5.1). Many observers felt it was time for a universal public program that offered special protections to these low-income beneficiaries.

Table 5.1 PROPORTION OF ELDERLY IN THE UNITED STATES WITH OUT-OF-POCKET SPENDING MORE THAN 15 PERCENT OF INCOME, BY INCOME AND HOSPITAL USE, 1986

Income	Proportion of Elderly Spending More than 15 Percent of Income		
	All Elderly (%)	Elderly with a Hospital Stay (%)	Elderly with No Hospital Stay (%)
All Incomes	23.9	39.9	19.5
$10,000 or Less	37.0	56.2	31.6
More than $10,000	5.6	16.2	2.8

Source: Feder et al. (1987b).

Setting the Stage for the Legislation

The Medicare Catastrophic Coverage Act owed its initial political impetus to the Bowen Commission—a group headed by former Secretary of Health and Human Services Otis Bowen. The Commission was charged by President Reagan with studying problems associated with catastrophic health expenses, including both acute- and long-term care for persons of all ages. Testimony to the commission stressed the critical need for long-term care protection for the elderly, in particular. But the Bowen report, released in fall 1986, only proposed legislation to deal with the problem of gaps in acute care for Medicare beneficiaries (U.S. Department of Health and Human Services 1987). This issue was viewed as the "easiest" to solve of the major healthcare access problems, because it was likely to be least expensive, requiring only marginal changes to address the problem.[2]

The original Bowen proposal called for a simple expansion of benefits financed with a flat $59 annual premium assessed on all Medicare enrollees. This was to be added to the existing Part B premium, fully covering the costs of the program. The benefit improvement would consist of an annual $2,000 limit on each beneficiary's out-of-pocket expenses arising from hospital and physician deductibles and coinsurance. Once the beneficiary paid $2,000, the Medicare program would forgive all further Medicare cost sharing under both Parts A and B in that calendar year, irrespective of beneficiary income and assets. In addition, hospital cost sharing would be limited to no more than two deductibles per year. Otherwise, Medicare would remain the same. This simple proposal added so-called stop-loss protection to Medicare similar to that found in many employer-covered policies.

EVOLUTION OF THE LEGISLATION

The willingness of the Reagan administration to support a $2 billion expansion in Medicare benefits took many by surprise. This legislation was proposed in 1986 at a time when previous annual budget submissions by the administration had routinely sought reductions in Medicare spending of at least that amount (e.g., Office of the President 1986). Not surprisingly, when the White House agreed to support the Bowen proposal, it did so with a number of stringent constraints attached—namely, that new benefits must be self-financed by the beneficiaries and that the financing must come from premiums paid by beneficiaries rather than from general taxes. The flat premium of about $5 per month that was part of the proposal was to be a straightforward increase in insurance coverage. Thus, although the bill would expand the scope of government benefits, it would not expand subsidies to elderly and disabled persons. In this sense, it was consistent with administration goals not to raise taxes—although it would still have expanded the scope of the federal government.

Despite initial concerns, Capitol Hill staff and lobbyists generally accepted the framework established by the Reagan administration as a starting point. But any hope that long-term care would be added by Congress was fleeting. Even the idea of a flat cap on spending as a desirable means for offering catastrophic protection went largely unchallenged, even though many in the research community had questioned the effectiveness of such caps in protecting lower-income beneficiaries, given differences in income (Berki 1986; Congressional Budget Office 1983; Feder et al. 1987b; Varner 1987; Wyszewianski 1986). Capitol Hill staffers and interest groups such as the AARP began to develop their own versions of legislation, but worked within the broad outlines of the Bowen proposal.

Within this framework, the contents of the benefit package were soon transformed. The Democrats in Congress, vowing not to be outdone by the Republicans in offering new legislation to expand Medicare, were handed a tough challenge: to enhance the benefits while keeping to the constraint of self-financing through premiums insisted upon by President Reagan. How much could be added without risking a presidential veto?

Defining the Benefits

During the spring of 1987, a number of modest additions to Bowen's package began to surface. For example, an early draft from the House Committee on Ways and Means added a limit on Part B out-of-pocket liabilities, simplified the hospital benefit, and improved coverage for home healthcare and skilled nursing facility (SNF) care. (As described in chapter 3, stringent regulations had restrained growth in the latter two benefits. Moreover, the requirement of three days' hospitalization before entering an SNF, as well as high coinsurance beginning on day 21 of a stay, also discouraged beneficiaries from claiming further benefits.)

Changes in home health and SNF care were viewed as minor improvements in the long-term care area. Even many supporters of publicly provided long-term care thought that a major move to include it in this legislation was too radical an addition to be feasible, largely because of its cost. When Congressman Claude Pepper tried to interest members in adding his home care bill to the package, there was strong opposition from all quarters.[3]

But as the spring progressed, two other broad additions were made by the House of Representatives. First, major Medicaid expansions were added to provide relief from Medicare coinsurance and deductibles for the low-income elderly, as well as to improve the financial protection of spouses of nursing home residents. The first of these changes required that the program pay Medicare coinsurance, deductibles, and premiums for all Medicare beneficiaries with incomes below poverty. (Less than half of poor Medicare recipients had Medicaid coverage in 1987, since states' eligibility standards for Medicaid were generally stringent.) This was a way to add further protections for low-income beneficiaries without differentiating coverage within the Medicare program itself. The approach recognized that a $2,000 cap on spending was too high to protect the poor from "unaffordable" healthcare costs, and since the change was to be added through Medicaid, it would not seem to be "means testing" the benefits.

The spousal impoverishment provisions raised the amount of income and assets a spouse could keep when the husband or wife received Medicaid support for nursing home expenses, thus increasing the number of people eligible for Medicaid.

These Medicaid provisions could effectively be funded with dollars freed up at the state level by other provisions in the legislation. That is, when Medicare's coverage became more generous with the stop-loss and other protections, Medicaid costs for persons already covered by both programs would fall and states' burdens for the over-65 population would be eased. By expanding Medicaid in this way, the MCCA sought to prevent states from reducing their own healthcare spending in response to the new provisions.[4]

The second major expansion added drug coverage to the package. In part, this was viewed as a way to offer benefits to higher-income enrollees who were being asked to pay a disproportionate share of the costs of the legislation (discussed in the following subsection). This change established an entirely new benefit. But to keep it a "catastrophic" benefit (i.e., restricted to those with well above average healthcare expenses), there would be a high deductible before Medicare would begin to pay. Even so, a substantial number of Medicare beneficiaries would qualify. Many advocates of this drug coverage expected older persons to view it as a major improvement in Medicare.

The Senate Committee on Finance proceeded more cautiously than the House, but within a very similar framework. Its final package looked like a scaled-down version of the House bill, but without the drug benefit.

The drug, SNF, home health, and Medicaid expansions added by the House of Representatives tripled the estimated costs of the MCCA. A July 1987 Congressional Budget Office study estimated the average annual benefits per enrollee at $78 for Bowen and $226 for the House version.

Financing

These benefit escalations created a major problem on the financing side. Although $5 per month might not be viewed as unduly burdensome on those with modest incomes, a $20 premium (added to the already escalating Part B premium) could hurt those it presumably sought to help: the low-income elderly, who had trouble buying private supplemental insurance and meeting high out-of-pocket healthcare costs. Some other means of financing the benefit became imperative.

Under the Ways and Means Committee proposal, everyone (except those covered by Medicaid) would pay a basic premium (of $31 annually in the first year). To this would be added a supplemental, income-related portion that would affect persons with adjusted gross incomes above $6,250, after which this supplemental premium would rise steeply to a maximum of $580 for those with adjusted gross incomes of $14,166 or more.[5] This produced a premium schedule that was only progressive for those with the lowest incomes. Medicare enrollees with as little as $20,000 in income would pay as much in total premiums as enrollees who were extremely wealthy. Wealthier elderly families would pay a smaller share of their incomes in supplemental premiums than middle-income beneficiaries—a regressive burden for those with incomes above $20,000.

The Senate addressed the issue quite differently, assessing a higher initial flat premium and then adding a supplemental premium that rose much more gradually by income. The maximum income-related premium was set at $800 per enrollee, but would apply only to beneficiaries with incomes over $60,000—making the Senate version more like a standard surtax on the income tax, rising gradually with income. Although it too would become regressive above about $60,000, many fewer Medicare beneficiaries have incomes above that level. Figure 5.1 compares the two approaches.

Figure 5.1 ADDITIONAL PREMIUMS UNDER SELECTED CATASTROPHIC PLANS
BY ADJUSTED GROSS INCOME, 1989

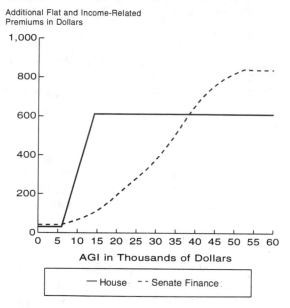

Source: Congressional Budget Office (1988).

The term *supplemental premium* was carefully chosen to distinguish it from a tax increase. It was to be administered through the Internal Revenue Service (IRS), however, and paid using the 1040 form, making it seem suspiciously like a tax. The House version was even mandatory. The Senate version had a greater claim to the term *premium*, since it proposed to treat this new benefit as a voluntary option. Beneficiaries could choose to enroll in the catastrophic benefit or to decline coverage. The actual choice turned out to be less voluntary than it might initially seem, however, since individuals would have to forgo *all* of the heavily subsidized Part B coverage if they opted out of catastrophic. In practice, few beneficiaries would be likely to opt out.

THE MEDICARE CATASTROPHIC COVERAGE ACT: PASSAGE AND REPEAL

When the Medicare Catastrophic Coverage Act was passed in June of 1988, it was hailed as "the largest expansion of Medicare since the

program's establishment in 1965" (Torres-Gil 1989). A major ceremony was held in the Rose Garden of the White House on July 1, 1988,
to celebrate its signing by President Ronald Reagan. In private, the
enthusiasm of the drafters was considerably lower—reflecting the long
road of compromises necessary to enact such legislation.

The final benefit package was a complex combination of fill-in and
new benefits that built on the House version, as summarized in table
5.2.

On the Part A side, the legislation reduced beneficiaries' liability
for hospital care to only one deductible per year. Beyond that, hospital
benefits would cover the full year, eliminating the concept of spell of
illness and all of the coinsurance calculations necessary under the
original program. This expansion and simplification of hospital coverage represented one of the more valuable benefit changes of the act;
these benefits became effective in January 1989.[6]

Also on the Part A side, the SNF benefit was made more generous
by eliminating the requirement of a 3-day prior hospital stay, by
lengthening the coverage to 150 days per year, and by reducing and
rearranging the coinsurance charged. Coinsurance would be required
for the first 8 days—but at a much lower rate of 20 percent of the daily
cost of nursing home care.[7] These changes meant that more beneficiaries would qualify for coverage and that longer stays would be covered. These changes also took force in 1989. In retrospect, SNF
changes (combined with some regulatory easing in 1988) turned out
to be more substantial than originally credited and would have made
important contributions to the costs of short nursing home stays over
time had the legislation not been repealed (Liu and Kenney 1991).

Hospice and home health benefits were also modestly expanded by
relaxing some of the requirements on participation in these areas. The
210-day lifetime limit on hospice benefits was eliminated. The home
health benefit was also made less restrictive by relaxing the intermittency standards. Enrollees would be able to receive up to 38 consecutive days of care, 7 days a week. (Interpretation of the original intermittency requirements had stated that visits could be no more
frequent than 5 days per week for no more than 3 consecutive weeks.)
Implementation of the home health changes was set to begin in 1990.

On the Part B side, the major expansion was a limit on the amount
of deductibles and copayments beneficiaries would pay for physician
and other services, for the first time placing a cap on how much
Medicare beneficiaries would have to pay out of pocket for Part B
coinsurance and deductibles. Above the cap, Medicare would pay the
full 100 percent of allowed charges.[8] This cap would have started at

Table 5.2 MEDICARE CATASTROPHIC COVERAGE ACT BENEFITS AS ENACTED IN 1988

1989	1990	1991	1992	1993
Hospital Insurance				
Hospital Inpatient Benefits. Provides unlimited inpatient hospital care. Eliminates all copayments and deductibles except one annual deductible amount ($560 in 1989).	**Home Health Benefits.** Relaxes current requirement that limits home healthcare to intermittent visits; enrollees may receive up to 38 consecutive days of care, seven days a week.	All hospital insurance benefits in place after 1990.		
Skilled Nursing Facility (SNF) Benefits. Increases limit on SNF stays to 150 days a year and requires no prior hospital stay. Coinsurance is required for first eight days each year, at 20 percent of average SNF costs per day ($25.50 for 1989).				
Hospice Benefits. Eliminates 210-day lifetime limit on hospice benefits, but retains a cost limit.				
Supplementary Medical Insurance (SMI)				
No provisions take effect in 1989.	**Limitation on Part B Cost Sharing.** Limits out-of-pocket expenses for covered Part B services ($1,370 in 1990). Adjusts the cap yearly to keep proportion of eligible enrollees constant at 7 percent.	All SMI provisions in place after 1990. **Limitation on Part B Cost Sharing.** Part B cap increases to $1,530.	**Limitation on Part B Cost Sharing.** Part B cap increases to $1,700.	**Limitation on Part B Cost Sharing.** Part B cap increases to $1,900.

Mammography. Expands coverage to include mammography screening.

Respite Care. Eighty percent of reasonable costs is paid for up to 80 hours a year of in-home personal services, to give homebound enrollees' usual caretakers a respite. Eligibility occurs after Part B copayment cap or prescription drug deduction is met.

Catastrophic Drug Insurance

No provisions take effect in 1989.

Limited Drug Benefits. Covers drugs administered intravenously at home, with a 20 percent coinsurance, and immuno-suppressive drugs, with a 20 percent coinsurance for the first year after transplant surgery (thereafter, the regular prescription drug coinsurance applies). Deductible in 1990, $550; coinsurance, 50 percent.

Full Drug Benefits. Covers all outpatient prescription drugs and insulin, subject to a deductible ($600 in 1991) that will be adjusted annually so the proportion of eligible enrollees will remain constant at 16.8 percent. Requires coinsurance of 50 percent of reasonable charges above the deductible in 1991.

Full Drug Benefits. Deductible, $652; coinsurance, 40 percent.

Full Drug Benefits. Deductible, $710; coinsurance falls to 20 percent in 1993 and subsequent years.

Source: ProPAC (1990).

$1,370 in 1990 and risen each year at a rate intended to protect the 7 percent of enrollees with the highest Part B costs. The main beneficiaries of this stop-loss would be persons with surgeries or other very expensive physician procedures.

The major new addition to Medicare services was the drug benefit, covering outpatient prescription drugs above a $600 deductible. This very large deductible was designed to limit this benefit to users with unusually high liabilities. The benefit was to phase in with only immunosuppressive drugs and intravenously administered drugs at home covered in 1990. Then in 1991, coverage was to expand to include all outpatient prescription drugs and insulin. Initially, enrollees would be required to pay coinsurance of 50 percent. That requirement would be reduced over time to a 20 percent coinsurance.

Finally, Part B was expanded to include biennial mammography screening and a small respite benefit. Medicare would pay up to 80 percent of reasonable costs for up to 80 hours a year of in-home personal services to provide relief to caregivers of homebound enrollees. The coverage would only be available to those exceeding either the Part B payment cap or the drug deductible, however. Thus, it was essentially a symbolic addition to Medicare's benefit package that would be available to only a small portion of enrollees.

The Medicaid changes previously mentioned were also part of the legislation. These changes added protections for low-income Medicare beneficiaries against Medicare cost sharing and premiums and raised the income and asset protections for the spouse left in the community.

The financing package reflected a compromise between the Senate and House provisions. The flat premium was smaller than under the Senate version, but the structure of the supplemental premium looked more like the Senate's more gradual rate of premium increases. The supplemental premium would be assessed against any beneficiary whose income tax liability was at least $150. Beginning in 1989, such individuals would pay at the rate of $22.50 per $150 in liability (effectively a 15 percent surtax). The maximum liability was set at $800 per enrollee; individuals with incomes of over about $40,000 would be subject to that maximum. Couples with incomes in excess of about $70,000 would pay $1,600. Estimates indicated that only about 5 percent of older persons would be subject to these maximum tax levels, and that about 40 percent of all the elderly would pay at least some supplemental premium. But this surtax rate would rise rapidly over time to a maximum of 28 percent by 1993, or nearly double the initial rate. Over time, a larger proportion of Medicare enrollees would pay this surtax.

Another important element of the financing was that the premiums were set to begin in 1989, whereas several of the key benefits were not scheduled to go into effect until later. Revenues would thus be considerably higher than outlays in the early years. This provision would allow for the buildup of reserves in a newly created trust fund, to ensure sufficient funds as new benefits came on line. It also had the short-run effect of reducing the federal deficit, and would later come under fire by beneficiaries suspicious of whether they were being taxed for new benefits or for deficit reductions.

Overall Beneficiary Impact

Altogether, these changes would have increased Medicare benefits per enrollee by about 7 percent. This estimate is based on a Congressional Budget Office simulation of the impact of the MCCA, on the assumption that all benefits were fully in place in 1988 (Christensen and Kasten 1988b). If so, catastrophic benefits would have averaged $194 per enrollee, yielding total Medicare benefits averaging $2,995 compared to $2,801 under "current law." Table 5.3 presents a breakdown of these components. Most (89 percent) of the $194 was due to reductions in the Medicare copayments. The rest represented new service use or relaxation of coverage limits.

The Medicaid buy-in would have reduced copayment liabilities by another $28 per beneficiary, averaged over the total enrollee population. For the much smaller number of elderly and disabled persons actually eligible for this buy-in, the benefits would have averaged $350 (Christensen and Kasten 1988a).

The CBO simulation also illustrates the relationship of these benefits to Medigap coverage. New Medicare benefits would reduce Medigap benefit payments by 25 percent, since Medicare is the first payer of services. The other 75 percent of the benefits paid by private insurers would remain as liabilities for Medicare beneficiaries—mainly Part B coinsurance up to the cap and the Part A and B deductibles. Medigap premiums would fall by about 20 percent in response to these changes—less of a reduction in premiums than the reduction in out-of-pocket payments policyholders would have to make.

Viewed in a different context, less than one-third of the benefits from the MCCA would overlap with services covered by Medigap insurance. Some of the difference reflects the fact that only about two-thirds of Medicare beneficiaries had Medigap coverage. But even for those with such coverage, over half the catastrophic benefits would exceed what private insurers cover. In other words, these new benefits

Table 5.3 MEDICARE BENEFIT PAYMENTS, COPAYMENT LIABILITIES, AND
PREMIUMS PAYABLE PER ENROLLEE BEFORE AND AFTER
IMPLEMENTATION OF MEDICARE CATASTROPHIC COVERAGE ACT OF
1988

	Before	After	Change
Medicare benefit payments per enrollee[a]			
Hospital Insurance	$1,693	$1,747	$ 54
Supplementary Medical Insurance	1,108	1,191	83
Catastrophic Drug Insurance	0	57	57
Total	2,801	2,995	194
Medicare copayment liabilities per enrollee			
Hospital Insurance	162	118	−44
Supplementary Medical Insurance	325	262	−63
Catastrophic Drug Insurance	244	179	−65
Total	731	559	−172
Medicare premiums payable per enrollee			
Monthly premiums	290	368	78
Supplemental premiums	0	129	129
Total	290	497	207

Source: Congressional Budget Office (1988).
Note: Table shows effects of Medicare only.
a. About 22 percent of enrollees were estimated to be entitled to higher Medicare benefit
payments under the MCCA when fully implemented. This reflects an unduplicated
count of those affected by the Hospital Insurance provisions (4 percent), the Supplementary Medical Insurance copayment cap (7 percent), and the drug provisions (16.8
percent).

would lower the out-of-pocket spending by Medicare beneficiaries,
but not eliminate the role of Medigap.

Winners and Losers

Proponents of the passage of catastrophic coverage believed they had
achieved a major improvement in benefits. For example, the largest
interest group representing the elderly, the AARP, enjoyed accolades
concerning the considerable role the organization had played in working with Congress on the MCCA (Torres-Gil 1989). Other organizations
of the elderly and organized labor had also worked hard to secure
passage.

The MCCA also had vehement opponents, however. The drug industry, fearing government interference in its activities, bitterly fought
inclusion of the drug benefit in the program. Although the industry
could not block the legislation, it managed to water down the drug

benefit provisions. For example, no reference was made in the legislation to any type of cost controls on drugs; instead, the final bill called for beneficiaries to pay higher premiums over time if costs exceeded expectations. The Pharmaceutical Manufacturers Association reportedly spent several million dollars to oppose the legislation and, failing that, to seek limitations on cost controls (Rich 1987). Some insurance companies in the Medigap field also actively opposed the legislation.

The National Committee to Preserve Social Security and Medicare, a latecomer to the debate, was also against the bill, seeking to derail the financing scheme and eliminate the supplemental premium. They mounted a major lobbying and letter-writing campaign that was unsuccessful, at least in part because their often deceptive mail campaigns were viewed by members of Congress more as a fundraising ploy than as legitimate grassroots organizing (Simon 1989). Opposition to the legislation from other seniors groups was only beginning to get organized when the legislation passed.

As noted, the final package was intended to be budget neutral from the federal government's perspective, although there were clearly individual winners and losers. On the benefit side, additional benefits directed at low-income beneficiaries through the Medicaid program assured that many low-income enrollees would be winners. Differences in the use of health services by various groups also meant that the level of benefits received varied in any given year. For example, the very old with high rates of hospital use were more likely to benefit than younger, healthier enrollees.

Table 5.4 displays the Congressional Budget Office's estimated insurance benefits (for just the Medicare portion of the MCCA) and costs in terms of premiums paid, by the income status of enrollees (Congressional Budget Office 1988), on the assumption of full implementation. Out-of-pocket costs for covered services would be lower for all income groups, but the cost reductions would increase steadily as the beneficiary group gets poorer. This redistribution would be even greater if the Medicaid changes targeted at low-income persons had been added to the table.

When the financing side is added in, the redistribution becomes much more dramatic. The bottom 70 percent of Medicare enrollees as ranked by their incomes would have a net reduction in out-of-pocket costs. On average, these enrollees would pay considerably less in premiums than they would, on average, gain in increased protections. The top 30 percent, in contrast, would face higher costs primarily because of the supplemental premium. If the table 5.4 estimates took

Table 5.4 NET CHANGE IN ENROLLEES' OUT-OF-POCKET COSTS BY INCOME
AND POVERTY STATUS IN RESPONSE TO MEDICARE CATASTROPHIC
COVERAGE ACT OF 1988

Enrollees' Income and Poverty Status	Percentage of Enrollees in Group	Net Change from[a]		
		Cost Sharing and New Benefits	Premium Increases	Total Impact
By Per Capita Income Percentiles (average per capita income)				
0 to 10 ($2,881)	10.0	$ − 237	$80	$ − 158
11 to 30 ($5,623)	20.0	− 221	81	− 140
31 to 50 ($8,575)	20.0	− 195	89	− 106
51 to 70 ($12,604)	20.0	− 189	157	− 32
71 to 90 ($19,579)	20.0	− 171	373	203
91 to 100 ($52,291)	10.0	− 161	597	436
By Poverty Status				
Poor	12.8	− 232	80	− 152
Near Poor[b]	19.4	− 226	79	− 147
Other	67.8	− 178	268	90
All enrollees	100.0	− 194	207	13

Source: Congressional Budget Office (1988).
a. Assumes full implementation in 1988. Includes only Medicare changes.
b. Includes those with incomes above poverty line but below 1.5 times the line.

into account whether certain groups already had private insurance protection (or whether that protection was provided free of charge to those whose former employers paid the costs), the redistribution would be still more dramatic since almost all high-income individuals have Medigap coverage and many of them have it subsidized or fully paid by their former employers. Such individuals would see few new benefits, only new costs.

A full understanding of the effects of the MCCA also requires appreciation that average effects for an income group hide differences within the group. First, the effects of healthcare change differ by gender and race. Women use relatively more long-term care and men relatively more acute care, implying that the MCCA would benefit men more than women. Black beneficiaries use less care than whites, because of both access constraints and low income. To the extent that the MCCA facilitated access, black beneficiaries would stand to gain more than their white counterparts. Disabled beneficiaries also use more Medicare services than their elderly nondisabled counterparts, implying that they would benefit more from the MCCA.

Second, how much any individual in a group would benefit relative to others in the same income or demographic group depends on actual healthcare use. Many beneficiaries could expect little change in their benefits unless they were hospitalized several times or for long periods, or unless they had very high expenses overall. It is the very nature of catastrophic protection that although the benefits can be substantial when triggered, very few individuals reach that category initially. Indeed, some of the benefits were defined to grow over time only enough to protect a certain percentage of all beneficiaries. The Congressional Budget Office (1988) estimated that when fully implemented the MCCA would provide some additional benefits to 22 percent of all beneficiaries in a given year. Cumulated over a longer period, more than 22 percent would receive direct benefits.

Third, other changes, although substantial for those who needed them, were limited to a small share of Medicare enrollees. For example, elimination of the hospital coinsurance requirements and lifting of the lifetime limits on hospitalization would each year affect only about 0.5 percent of all enrollees, about 165,000 persons. But for those individuals with extremely heavy healthcare burdens, the benefits would be substantial.

Many opponents of the legislation used the relatively small numbers of persons who would *directly* receive help in any given year to argue that the MCCA was a "bad deal." They ignored the fact that everyone with the new coverage would gain needed protection whether or not they actually need to use it, because all of them are at risk. This is the principle of catastrophic coverage.

The Beginning of the End

The subsequent debate made it abundantly clear that beneficiaries as a group either did not understand that fundamental principle or did not value such protection very highly. Even after passage of the MCCA in 1988, opponents—led by the Pharmaceutical Manufacturers Association and the National Committee to Preserve Social Security and Medicare—kept up a steady barrage of protest and captured considerable media attention. Those in Congress who had opposed the legislation from the beginning played to this protest.

Two sets of information fed this opposition. First came word in the spring of 1989 that the U.S. Treasury expected tax collections from the supplemental premium on the elderly to be higher than anticipated, generating a considerable buildup in the Catastrophic Coverage trust fund. Although some buildup had been intended in the legislation to provide a cushion for the benefits that would be phased in later but then would grow very rapidly, the Treasury Department's estimate of the size of the reserves was considerably higher than the level originally intended. Critics claimed that the new legislation was deliberately aimed at reducing the deficit at the expense of the elderly.

Senator Lloyd Bentsen, of Texas, already under pressure from his constitutents, announced on April 20, 1989, that he would seek a reduction in the supplemental premium to counteract the unexpected surplus. This promise captured considerable media attention. Other legislators generally took a more cautious approach, although they recognized the considerable pressure building on the supplemental premium.

Shortly therafter, however, the Congressional Budget Office released a second set of numbers indicating that the costs of some benefits had been severely underestimated. In particular, the improvements in the SNF benefit were now projected to cost more than six times the original estimate. One of the earliest provisions to be implemented, SNF use rose dramatically in early 1989. Between 1988 and 1989, covered days per stay jumped to 34 from 27, on average, representing a 26 percent increase in length of stay in just one year. And the number of persons covered rose from 392,438 in 1988 to 591,281 in 1989, largely as a result of eliminating the three-day prior hospital stay requirement (HCFA 1991, unpublished data).

The MCCA effectively allowed states to shift patients from Medicaid to Medicare. States took advantage of this change. Since this affected patients already in the system, even with no new admissions, Medicare costs would rise as existing patients were shifted from Medicaid to Medicare. The effect was exacerbated by nursing homes that previously had not found it in their interest to participate in Medicare beginning to participate, increasing the number of available SNF beds. The total number of SNF-covered days rose to over 25 million in 1989, nearly triple the amount for 1988 (Ways and Means 1991).[9]

In addition, the reestimates of the costs of the drug benefit—using newly available data—proved twice as high as the original figure (Congressional Budget Office 1989a). In this case, the change in the cost estimate resulted from the release of 1987 data showing a much greater jump in the use of drugs before the MCCA than the Congressional Budget Office had projected using older data. CBO had originally estimated spending growth per enrollee on drugs at an annual rate of 10 percent in the 1980s. The new data indicated that the rate between 1980 and 1987 had been over 14 percent per year. Thus, the projected value of the drug benefit to Medicare enrollees increased dramatically, creating a further expected drain on the revenues.

These new figures not only eliminated any surplus in the trust funds for a rollback of the supplemental premium, but projected a revenue shortfall. Senator Bentsen and others who had backed a roll-back in the supplemental premium were left hanging.

Although neither of these new data releases was politically moti-vated, their timing had a drastic political effect. In retrospect at least, the disappearance of the promised surplus, and with it the opportu-nity to roll back the supplementary premium—combined with the prospect of costs outstripping even the revenues that would be pro-duced by the "high" premium level—set the stage for eventual repeal as early as the spring of 1989. But the Senate and the House leadership resisted any immediate reconsideration of the legislation and many observers expected the furor to fade.

Such was not to be the case. Continued pressure of the mail cam-paigns launched by well-funded opponents[10] and the generally nega-tive tone of the media began to take their toll.

A major blow came in the late summer of 1989. Those who stood to benefit from the MCCA had remained silent since its passage. But a vocal minority made its protest heard in town meetings held by members of Congress in their home districts. The most dramatic of these saw a confrontation with Congressman Dan Rostenkowski that made the national news over Labor Day weekend. A number of elderly protestors blocked Rostenkowski's departure from a town meeting in Illinois. Captured on camera was an elderly woman pounding the hood of the car while the driver attempted to move through the crowd. Eventually, Rostenkowski "fled" on foot from view of CNN cameras. For all the world to see, an opponent of the legislation had "sent a message" to the chairman of the most powerful committee in the House of Representatives. It no longer mattered that these protesters represented only a minority of the elderly—they were vocal, visible, and seemingly growing stronger by the day.

Repeal

Even before the August recess, an earnest effort was begun in Congress to modify the Catastrophic legislation. As the hope of proponents that the protest would prove short-lived died, congressional committees began to search for a compromise to save at least part of the legislation. Although some of the interest groups, such as the National Committee to Preserve Social Security and Medicare, argued to keep all the benefits while changing the financing, most of the effort centered on what benefits could be retained if the supplemental premium were eliminated. There was little serious discussion of adding additional revenue sources: the original agreement to stick with a self-financed benefit package remained intact. The difficulty lay in deciding which benefits were the most important. Each had proponents who had worked within the legislative framework during passage and who felt they had already compromised enough.

Many options were proposed, but none seemed to capture the imagination of enough members of Congress to go anywhere. A number of those leading the charge for repeal had been opposed to the legislation from the start, so they were unlikely to ally themselves with supporters in a compromise. One of the last objections to repeal was that it would count against (and thus increase) the federal deficit. Despite the lip service paid to supporting the MCCA by the Bush administration, the Office of Management and Budget (OMB) indicated that an exception would be granted so that repeal would not be so counted.[11] The death knell had sounded.

On October 4, 1989, the House of Representatives voted for repeal of all but the Medicaid provisions. The Senate passed an amendment to salvage at least some of the benefits while eliminating the dreaded supplemental premium. However, the Senate's amendment was rejected by the House. On the last night of the session, members of the House, who literally sat with their coats on their laps, considered and then rejected it. The Senate followed suit and voted repeal of all but the Medicaid low-income benefits. In the early hours of November 22, 1989, the U.S. Congress took the nearly unprecedented step of repealing a major piece of social legislation only one year after passage.

LESSONS FOR HEALTH POLICY

The issues surrounding this extraordinary turn of events and their implications for future health policy will be debated for years to come. Several lessons are already clear. Some are insights into the political process. Others are lessons for Medicare's future.

Politics of the Supplemental Premium

More than any other element of the legislation, beneficiaries objected to the supplemental premium. Medicare's Part B premium had always been a flat payment assessed on everyone except the very poorest beneficiaries, who are also covered by Medicaid. The new financing was a dramatic departure. For the first time, Medicare differentiated among beneficiaries, and at its apex, the supplemental premium represented an enormous increase in beneficiary contributions.

Scare Tactics That Worked

Although only a small share of beneficiaries—about 5 percent—would actually have had to pay the maximum supplemental amount, much of the publicity generated by groups supporting repeal were successful in suggesting otherwise. For example, one flyer produced by a group calling itself the Seniors Coalition Against the Tax asked in bold letters: "Will you get an $800 tax bill for Catastrophic coverage this year?" Its readers were not invited to think there might be more than one answer. Even among beneficiaries who understood perfectly well that they would not have to pay the maximum, opponents were able to stimulate objections to the principle—and the precedent—that *anyone* on Medicare would have to pay such a sum.

The supplemental premium was developed by the House Ways and Means Committee as a way to meet the Reagan administration's requirement that there should be no new taxes and that any financing should come from the beneficiaries themselves. The inevitable result of this requirement was a large premium on middle- and high-income beneficiaries. At a top supplemental premium of $800 plus the flat premium of $48, the highest-income beneficiaries would have paid nearly four times the actuarial value of their expected new benefits. And even with such a high maximum, it was still necessary to phase in the supplemental premium on middle-income beneficiaries to raise enough revenue. Moreover, this amount was projected to grow rapidly, reaching a maximum combined premium of $1,172 by 1993—equivalent to a surtax of 28 percent on top of other income tax liabilities (Congressional Budget Office 1988).

Current law at that time required beneficiaries to pay only 25 percent of the costs of Part B. The MCCA would have raised this share for the highest-income beneficiaries to about 75 percent of the overall costs of their Part B coverage (Christensen and Kasten 1988a). This would still have been a subsidy, of course, but not a very attractive alternative to beneficiaries who had been enjoying a far more generous subsidy out of general revenues for many years.

SEMANTICS THAT BACKFIRED

Throughout the debate, both Congress and the organizations supporting the legislation took care to retain the nomenclature of supplemental premium to distinguish it from a "tax." But it was to be collected by the IRS through the regular income tax structure and calculated on the basis of how much income tax a beneficiary owed, just like a surtax. Martin Corry, chief lobbyist for the AARP, was quoted as saying the IRS was involved "simply [as] an administrative convenience. It just happens to be the most efficient way of handling it" (Rich 1988). Such pronouncements did not prevent the beneficiaries from seeing it as a surtax. Worse, the semantic distinction was widely perceived as disingenuous if not dishonest.

The situation was made worse by the litany of the Reagan administration that no one should have to pay more taxes. The trend in the 1980s, indeed, had been to lower personal income tax rates. A perceived exception that singled out the elderly and disabled seemed a particularly glaring exception. Terming it the "seniors' tax" (or even the "AARP tax") enabled opponents to portray the financing of the MCCA in a very negative light. Further, higher income beneficiaries were being asked to pay more than a dollar for a dollar's worth of additional benefits when we were financing the rest of the budget with 85 cents of taxes and 15 cents in borrowing for each dollar spent.

A LOPSIDED DEBATE

The linking of a financing mechanism to new program benefits in this highly visible way reflected the philosophy of Congress and the administration that no new spending should worsen the deficit. It reflected more—that the additional revenues be found from within the program itself. The MCCA went even further, creating a reserve in a new trust fund to ensure that benefits would not exceed revenues.

As it turned out, objections to the "tax" swamped discussion of the benefits. Was this a specific reaction to the MCCA? Or does it raise wider issues about a legislative approach that links the two so closely and inextricably? It is too soon to judge the long-term consequences of requiring such pairing of benefits and financing, but this episode does suggest that any social legislation seeking to help one group through payment levied on another group within the same program may face formidable obstacles to achieving success.

The Reagan administration did not help itself in this respect with its repeated assertion that tax increases were unnecessary and that government could be financed and savings obtained simply by cutting fat out of the system. Its rhetoric worked against it in trying to secure acceptance of the MCCA—its only major piece of social legislation in either term.

Lessons for Medicare's Future

Perhaps more important than any political lessons are the lessons we can learn from the MCCA for Medicare's future. Indeed, the ultimate outcome for Medicare in the 1990s may well be to embrace the very parts of the MCCA that helped contribute to its demise.

BENEFIT PACKAGE DESIGN

The final MCCA legislation offered net benefit increases to the vast majority of Medicare beneficiaries. But these were typically modest and came in a bewildering variety of forms. Changes occurred in at least eight areas: hospital care, skilled nursing care, home healthcare, a Part B limit on copayments, hospice, respite care, mammograms, and drugs. All but the first made the already Byzantine Medicare program even more complex. Most beneficiaries did not understand how the existing benefit package worked. How were they supposed to interpret the changes? Interpretation was not helped by the fact that each of the new benefits was small and that together they averaged only a little over $200 per beneficiary per year—large enough to cause financing difficulties for a program as large as Medicare but hard to sell as a substantial improvement in benefits.

There was no consistent theme or logic to the many disparate changes in the MCCA, making the whole somehow seem less than the sum of its parts. Since many older citizens focused much of their dissatisfaction with Medicare on the lack of long-term care benefits, a package of benefits built around long-term care as a theme might also have fared better. For example, incorporating Medicaid's spousal protection and the SNF and home care changes, and adding some further expansion of home care could have been packaged and sold as a first step toward long-term care—and perhaps for not much more than the cost of the MCCA if some restrictions were put on the benefits. Such a package would have been similar to the Pepper bill introduced a year later—which received relatively favorable reviews from seniors although it ran into trouble on the financing side. Ironically, the SNF benefit in the MCCA did turn out to be more significant than anticipated. But although the cost increases that it signaled were seized on by critics, the benefits for elderly and disabled persons went relatively unnoticed. A long-term care theme might have remedied that imbalance.

Catastrophic coverage itself can be a hard sell because, by definition, only a small proportion of enrollees will have occasion to use the benefits. Health policy experts agreed that the MCCA provisions were needed additions to the Medicare package—providing protection that was missing and offering relief to persons facing the danger of financial catastrophe because they have no supplemental coverage. But the average beneficiary did not see it that way. And given the particular design of the added protection within the Medicare context, they had a point.

The irony of the MCCA as finally passed was that its Medicare portion did not provide truly "catastrophic" protection for the low-income elderly or an attractive catastrophic alternative to those who could afford Medigap protection. And this fact highlights one of the major design challenges of providing catastrophic protection within the Medicare program. Since meaningful catastrophic protection depends on the income levels of those being covered, it is hard to think of an effective solution that is not means tested in some way. A $2,000 limit on out-of-pocket spending is valuable for someone with $30,000 of income, for example, but not for someone whose income is $5,000 or even $10,000. That person will stop being able to afford healthcare long before he or she has spent $2,000 on it, in order to pay for food and shelter. The healthcare catastrophe will have occurred long before the so-called catastrophic protection kicks in (Feder et al. 1987b). In this sense, the QMB protections that survived as a Medicaid change are a better approach.

And for beneficiaries well enough off for the $2,000 limit to be relevant, private Medigap protection was often a superior alternative to the MCCA protection. Such individuals could afford to purchase private catastrophic protection that was more generous—lower out-of-pocket caps and better first-dollar coverage—particularly when compared to the level of the supplemental premium. The MCCA coverage would have been more socially efficient (more comprehensive, less duplicative, and without the built-in incentive to use care that comes with first-dollar coverage). But those attributes were cold comfort to the higher-income beneficiaries who were paying more than the actuarial cost of the additional coverage.

RELATIONSHIP TO PRIVATE COVERAGE

As the foregoing discussion makes clear, the elderly as a whole were quite satisfied with Medigap coverage, voting with their wallets to continue it. The existence of Medigap policy allowed policyholders to choose different combinations of benefits. It also allowed them to continue any relationship they may have had with an insurance company before they became eligible for Medicare. Moreover, a substantial minority of elderly beneficiaries have their supplemental insurance paid for by a third party—usually an employer or former employer—typically providing rich benefit packages, including drug coverage. These are the beneficiaries who would have paid the $800 supplemental premium. Not only would their tax bite have risen, but they could legitimately claim they would benefit little from the MCCA.

Except for this high-income minority, however, as health experts pointed out, Medigap was not as efficient or all-encompassing as many of the elderly believed. As already noted, most Medigap policies do not provide as comprehensive coverage as the MCCA would have done. Only one-third of the MCCA's benefits in fact would have overlapped with benefits already covered by Medigap (Christensen and Kasten 1988a). This information was not widely known, and certainly not understood, by most Medicare enrollees.

Nor did they understand that much of the reimbursement they received for their Medicare-covered services was in fact paid by Medicare, not by Medigap. This is because statements about Medicare payments are forwarded to beneficiaries via the private insurance companies that process the claims. These are often the same companies that offer Medigap coverage. When Medicare is the first payer— as it is for most beneficiaries—Medicare's share is generally three to four times that of the Medigap company.

Proponents of the MCCA had assumed that the elderly would be glad to have the MCCA coverage, even if Medigap was currently covering it, because they would have appreciated the reduced premiums that would come from dropping the duplicative services. But the elderly simply did not hear, or if they heard they did not believe, the truth—that the MCCA coverage was more efficient for the vast majority of Medicare enrollees than the Medigap alternative.[12]

EFFECTS OF CHANGE ON SYSTEM COMPLEXITY

One factor never seriously addressed in the legislative debate over the MCCA changes was whether they added to the complexity of the Medicare program. Yet Medicare's complexity represents one of the long-standing complaints of beneficiaries. Medicare communications from HCFA are confusing and obscure, and it is difficult to know what benefits one has and what restrictions will affect them. The benefit package under the MCCA was almost assured of being undervalued, irrespective of any other factor, because of the complexity it added to the system.

As noted previously, the changes in the hospital coverage were the single exception. But since these represented only a fraction of the many changes, they seemed to get lost in the shuffle. They were also duplicative of the hospital cost-sharing benefit that almost every Medicare enrollee with any private coverage had as part of a Medigap policy.

The Part B cap and the drug benefit were both major benefits, but they sounded complicated and restrictive. The Part B cap offered an upper bound on liability (but only for formal Medicare cost sharing); the drug benefit required a substantial deductible. If it had been possible to tell beneficiaries that they would have to pay no more than, say, $2,000 or $3,000 out of pocket for hospital, physician, and drug expenses no matter what happened, the package might have been more understandable. But there were exceptions to the Part B cap, and drugs did not have any overall limit. Thus, even the notion of a "catastrophic cap" got lost in the mix of all the various pieces of the benefit.

The remaining benefits were more minor parts of Medicare—although as noted previously, the SNF expansion would have been more extensive than originally anticipated. Nonetheless, all of these benefits continued to have restrictions and limitations designed to keep them from being too expensive. As a consequence, they were dismissed by beneficiaries as too confusing or inapplicable to their situation.

MAKING DISTINCTIONS AMONG THE ELDERLY

Part of the significance of the MCCA was that it reflected a changing attitude toward America's elderly. No longer did members of Congress view persons over age 65 as a homogeneous group in need of public support. The financing mechanism of the act alone represented a formal acknowledgment of the disparities in economic status of the elderly. Under the MCCA, the most affluent of the elderly were not seen as deserving beneficiaries of an expanded Medicare program, but rather as the source of financing benefits for others. This major change in attitude stood in stark contrast to the views expressed when Medicare was first passed in 1965. During that debate, a generation earlier, the issue of means testing of Medicare also arose. But it was finessed by arguments that nearly all the elderly needed the health benefits and were too poor to buy them on their own (Marmor 1970). The higher average incomes of older persons made such an argument much harder to support in the 1980s. The MCCA thus signaled public recognition that policy may need to differentiate groups within the elderly.

Elderly Americans themselves, however, have resisted changes that would differentiate their ranks. Either because they reject the necessity of such a policy or perhaps because they understand its implications, older persons have sought to have Medicare remain a universal program with no distinctions by economic status or other characteristics. This may have benefited them so far, given the popularity of universal programs as compared to means-tested ones. But the issue is not going to disappear.

The MCCA was the first salvo in a potentially long and bitter debate over a changing view of older persons. Perhaps one of the greatest tactical mistakes of the MCCA's proponents was in moving too fast to differentiate treatment of beneficiaries. It is one thing to gradually introduce income-related premiums for Medicare and quite another to make the first step an $848 maximum premium tied to a benefit with an actuarial value of $250—plus benefits that many already claimed from other sources.

Both sides in the debate are now on the alert, hardening their respective positions. This issue pits people against each other in unusual ways. For example, relating benefits to income offers one way to substantially scale back the Medicare program for those who oppose the size of government. Indeed, an income-related premium for very high-income persons was proposed by the Bush administration in its fiscal 1993 budget submission (Office of the President 1992). But some supporters of elderly and disabled people see income-related premiums as a way to protect the most vulnerable, with perhaps no overall cut in the size of the program. The contradictory goals of these two groups, each of which supports income-related premiums for Medicare, make for strange political posturing.

CONCLUSIONS

The MCCA provided real benefits for a majority of older Americans and filled important gaps in the Medicare program. The simplification of Part A hospital benefits, the introduction of drug and respite benefits (even if quite limited), and the major and underestimated increase in the skilled nursing benefit would have wrought improvements in the healthcare coverage of older persons. Even many of those who already had Medigap coverage were likely to benefit. But the full measure of these improvements was not communicated well to beneficiaries.

It is, however, too easy to simply argue that older persons were misinformed. Analysts and policymakers ignored information that should have signaled problems. For years, older persons have demonstrated how much they like and are satisfied with the private supplemental policies that have grown up around Medicare. Displacing coverage that these policies now provide was not popular, and analysts could have anticipated that fact. Further, we have long known that universal programs enjoy much greater popularity in the United States than do means-tested ones. But the MCCA moved to change that formula, not to achieve major new benefits but to add marginal ones. The dramatic shift in the financing of Medicare was meaningful beyond the dollar value of the burden of the supplemental premium— it was a course change for Medicare that alarmed and angered many senior citizens. Fair or not, this was resented by many—even by those older persons who would have paid low premiums.

The MCCA also highlighted four important dilemmas that will continue to face health policy in the 1990s. First, it is expensive to make even minor expansions in large programs without large cost increases. Just adding $100 worth of new benefits means $3.8 billion in new costs, and these days, $100 buys relatively little healthcare. Second, individuals' perceptions of the value of such benefits lag behind their costs, resulting in sticker shock on the part of consumers and taxpayers. The value of these benefits was discounted by Medicare enrollees, but in truth, the average taxes that had to be raised were equivalent to the costs of the benefits. Third, a flat catastrophic cap set low enough to help those with low and modest incomes is very expensive, and not as generous as higher-income individuals could afford. Low-income persons need more help than we as a society feel we can afford for all beneficiaries in this era of fiscal stringency. Fourth, recognition of the varying economic circumstances of Medicare beneficiaries creates challenges to find a means to adapt the program to the needs of those who are still vulnerable without undermining strong public support for Medicare.

The repeal of the MCCA did not mean the end of changes in Medicare. The 1990s and beyond will continue to present many challenges for the program, challenges that can be faced intelligently only with knowledge of the lessons that the MCCA offers.

Notes

1. Gramm-Rudman-Hollings was an attempt by Congress to limit the size of the annual budget deficit and required across-the-board cutbacks in many federal programs if federal spending was projected to exceed certain targets.

2. Dealing with long-term care or the uninsured under age 65 would necessarily require large infusions of new public monies, so these areas were not seriously examined. The report did make some suggestions for expansion of private long-term care insurance.

3. The Pepper bill would have added a Part C to Medicare to cover supportive home care services under Medicare for both the current elderly and disabled population and for children under age 18. Congressman Pepper had also proposed to expand other services and to pay for these expansions with increased premiums and a higher limit on wages subject to the payroll tax (Varner 1987).

4. Not all these expanded benefits would go to the elderly and disabled populations; the MCCA also mandated some expansion in benefits for pregnant women and children.

5. Adjusted gross income (AGI) is a term used by the Internal Revenue Service for a particular line on the 1040 form. It is income after exemptions such as income from state and local bonds and the nontaxable portion of Social Security, but before deductions and personal exemptions.

6. Before passage, Medicare hospital benefits were defined around a spell-of-illness concept. For each spell of illness a beneficiary would have to pay the deductible, which could mean multiple payments in a given year. Moreover, benefits were limited to 60 days without any coinsurance. After that, coinsurance would be charged; after exhausting both the benefits within a spell of illness and the lifetime reserve days that could be added at the end of a spell, the beneficiaries would be liable for all further hospital charges themselves. (This is discussed in more detail in the appendix at the end of this volume.)

7. Previously, the coinsurance rate was tied to the hospital deductible, and the amount was higher, on average, than the full daily cost in many areas of the country.

8. Balance billing was not affected by the legislation and would not have counted toward the cap.

9. This change in SNF use was likely more dramatic than was expected from most of the other changes, because SNF use had for so long been very constrained. But even though this was likely the exception, it seemed to indicate the explosive nature of the expansion.

10. Among such opponents were the Pharmaceutical Manufacturers Association and some seniors' groups, particularly the National Committee to Preserve Social Security and Medicare and several smaller groups sometimes funded by drug companies. These more formal groups helped to mobilize the opposition, and in some cases spread a considerable amount of misleading information.

11. This was a technical issue. Because the MCCA created a trust fund that would help the federal deficit in the early years while it was building up, repeal of the MCCA would have had the unusual impact of temporarily *increasing* the federal deficit. Without this OMB exception, to remain budget neutral, taxes would have had to be raised to fund repeal of the legislation.

12. Well over 90 percent of all dollars spent on Medicare represent benefit payments to enrollees. For private insurance, average Medigap benefit payments per dollar of premium can be as low as 50 percent or 60 percent and seldom rise much above 80 percent to 85 percent (U.S. General Accounting Office 1991b).

Chapter Six

MARGINAL CHANGES AND THE FUTURE

The late 1990s are unlikely to be a period of business as usual for Medicare or the healthcare system in general. Medicare is sometimes cited as a model by supporters of national health insurance and many parts of it work well. But cries for reforms of all types swirl around the program. Some of these proposals advocate major restructuring of Medicare, often with an eye to fixing the fiscal problems that Part A will confront after the turn of the century, either as part of broader health reform, or more recently as simply a means for reducing federal spending. More extensive proposals are taken up in chapters 7 and 8. This chapter explores more marginal options for change that could be enacted in the absence of other reform in the healthcare system and that make sense even if the overall level of spending changes little.

RESTRUCTURING COST SHARING

The combination of deductibles and coinsurance for Medicare represents an ad hoc collection of payments with little justification as points of control for the use of healthcare services. When Medicare was introduced, the deductibles for Part A and Part B were set at nearly the same level: $40 and $50, respectively. But over time the Part A deductible has grown enormously—to $736 in 1996, compared to just $100 for Part B. Home health benefits required a coinsurance payment that was eliminated in 1973. But coinsurance for skilled nursing facility (SNF) benefits is at $92 a day, an amount well above the 20 percent established for other services. Thus, it makes sense to consider reshaping Medicare's cost sharing even in the absence of any larger effort to expand or contract the size of the Medicare program.

The goal of cost sharing is to provide cost awareness and thus give beneficiaries incentives to make careful use of services. But the importance of these incentives varies by type of healthcare service. In

Medicare, the most likely areas for expanding cost sharing to achieve appropriate service use are adding coinsurance for home health services and increasing the Part B deductible. More and more enrollees exceed the Part B deductible each year, since it has not kept up with Part B spending. It could be raised to $250 or $300 per year and still be comparable to or lower than that found in many private insurance plans. A second area for possible expansion would be home health coinsurance, although that would be a more controversial proposal, since this is a benefit used only by the very old and frail. After the coinsurance requirement for home health was eliminated in 1973, use of that benefit grew rapidly, particularly on the Part A side of Medicare (Kenney 1991). Some health analysts conclude that limited coinsurance might be a reasonable tool for moderating use of home health services (Moon et al. 1995).

Medicare's hospital and SNF cost sharing, in contrast, is already high. If cost sharing is used as more than just a tool for passing on a greater share of the costs to beneficiaries, some reductions in Part A cost sharing may also be appropriate. In practice, few advocates of cost sharing argue that hospital deductibles or coinsurance succeed in discouraging overuse of services. Patients rarely make the decision to check in to a hospital on their own. Moreover, there are other constraints on use of hospital care, such as preadmission screening, that serve to limit inappropriate use. And in the case of current coinsurance requirements for very long stays, hospitals themselves now have strong incentives to release their patients as early as possible because of incentives established by the Prospective Payment System (PPS). Consequently, hospital cost sharing could be substantially reduced with little or no expected increase in service use. In practice, however, hospital cost sharing requirements save the federal government considerable amounts (about $8 billion in 1996 by shifting costs onto beneficiaries and/or employers who help pay a share of retirees' health insurance (*Federal Register* 1995).

Another area of high cost sharing is the coinsurance on skilled nursing facility services. SNF coinsurance is out of line with the daily costs of such services since its rate is tied not to the costs of skilled nursing care but to the hospital deductible. This results in a benefit that appears to last 100 days, but which, for all practical purposes, loses much of its value to beneficiaries after just 20 days. Coinsurance on skilled nursing care will raise about $2 billion in 1996—and actually save considerably more than that in federal dollars, since it discourages use of this Medicare service.

Restructuring cost sharing could improve the Medicare program by shifting cost sharing to those areas where the incentives might be more effective, while simplifying the program. The reductions in cost sharing need to occur under Part A. If done in conjunction with an increase in cost sharing under Part B, the changes could be budget neutral overall. But this creates an issue within Medicare, since the two parts of the program are now financed separately and the Part A trust fund is in serious financial shape. A number of solutions are possible, including merging Parts A and B to create a single trust fund—a proposal that has often been made for Medicare but never enacted.[2]

A number of different combinations of cost sharing are possible that would remain revenue neutral (see table 6.1). Under each of the

Table 6.1 BUDGET NEUTRAL OPTIONS FOR RESTRUCTURING COST SHARING OF MEDICARE

		Part A				Part B
		Coinsurance				
Option	Hospital Deductible	Hospital	SNF	Home Health	Deductible	Monthly Premium
Current Law 1996	$736 for each spell of illness	$184 for days 61–90; $368 for days 91–150	$92 for days 21–100	None	$100	$42.50
1	$736 for first stay only	None	20% for days 21–100	Current law	$300	Current law
2	$500 for first stay only	None	20% for days 1–100	Current law	$350	Current law
3	$736 for first stay only	None	10% for days 1–100	Current law	$200	$50
4	$500 for first stay only	None	20% for days 21–100	Current law	$700, with Part A cost sharing counting toward cap	Current law

Source: Author's simulations using 1987 National Medical Expenditure Survey data, Congressional Budget Office 1992, and Federal Register 1995.
Note: Table assumes changes are fully implemented in 1996.

options shown, both the hospital coinsurance and the concept of a spell of illness would be eliminated. Beneficiaries would be covered for up to 365 days of hospital care. In each of these options, the SNF coinsurance would also be tied to the cost of SNF care; 20 percent coinsurance would be about $40 per day in 1996—a substantial reduction from its current $92 level. Most of the variation occurs in how the two deductibles would change. The more the hospital deductible is reduced, the higher the Part B deductible would need to be to keep the changes budget neutral. Option 3 in the table also funds part of the reduced cost sharing with a premium increase. Option 4 assumes that the Part B deductible would take into account Part A cost sharing, so that no beneficiary would face a deductible greater than $700 in total.

Each of these options would create different winners and losers. For example, option 4 in table 6.1 would mean that an individual with a hospital stay would only be subjected to a $200 deductible for Part B services ($700 minus $500); an individual without such a stay would not receive Medicare benefits until receiving over $700 in physician and related services. These two individuals would face a considerably different situation under option 1. A beneficiary with a hospital stay would prefer option 4 to the situation in option 1 in which he or she would face a $736 liability for the hospital stay and another $300 in physician services before Medicare began to pay. The individual without the hospital stay would be better off under option 1, where he or she would be subject to only a $300 deductible. Option 3 is similar to option 1 but reduces liabilities for those with long skilled nursing stays. In addition, instead of raising the Part B deductible substantially, option 3 relies on a modest increase plus a higher Part B premium.

COST-CONTAINMENT STRATEGIES

Since Medicare now constitutes nearly 10.5 percent of the federal budget (Office of the President 1996), it is likely to remain a target of budget reduction exercises for as long as the deficit remains a problem. As stated earlier, in each year of the Reagan and Bush administrations, the February budget submission to Congress called for substantial cuts in Medicare. The 1993 budget reduction bill put together by the Clinton administration resulted in $56 billion in savings from Medicare over five years. And in 1995, the Republican-led Congress proposed

$226 billion in savings over seven years and the Clinton administration countered with savings of $97 billion (Moon 1996). As yet, the debate on fiscal year 1996 spending and beyond remains unresolved even as the 1997 fiscal year budget—with $124 billion in Medicare reductions—was offered by the administration and rejected.

Ironically, although many politicians talk as though Social Security were an untouchable item in the budget, they do not seem to hold the same fear of tinkering with Medicare. Why is this so? A major explanation rests with the claim that most of the cuts are aimed at provider payments, moves that generally are viewed sympathetically by the elderly and disabled and their interest groups. Indeed, a slogan of the AARP about its approach to healthcare policy has been "Cut the Costs, Keep the Care." Many beneficiaries believe that hospitals and doctors are well paid for their services and sympathize with the calls for further belt-tightening. And Republican ads in 1995 suggested that most of the changes would come from attacking fraud and abuse, for example. The perception, then, is that cuts can be made without a direct reduction in benefits, unlike the case with Social Security. But as was emphasized in chapter 4, the cuts in Medicare have by no means been confined to providers, and even when they have been, such changes can have repercussions for beneficiaries as well. As this becomes more apparent with further provider restrictions, cost-containment efforts may meet more opposition. Indeed, part of the budget stalemate in 1995 reflected concerns about the public disapproval of some of the proposed Medicare changes.

Medicare is also more of a target than Social Security because Medicare is rising so fast that even substantive reductions in program generosity only help to slow its rate of growth. Further, even apart from the rest of the budget, lawmakers may be concerned with the continued financial viability of the program, since Part A is scheduled to face a financing crisis early in the next century.

One can safely predict that there will be continuing rounds of cost-containment activities directed at providers. Changes in provider payments constituted nearly two-thirds of the savings in the vetoed Balanced Budget Act of 1995, for example (Moon 1996). But such changes will not be enough to solve all of Medicare's financing problems even over the next decade. Instead, both restructuring of the program and increased beneficiary burdens are likely to be considered. The rest of this chapter considers relatively marginal changes that could take place to achieve savings. More radical restructuring is considered in chapter 7.

Hospitals

Across-the-board cuts in payments to hospitals for inpatient services served as the most fruitful area for achieving Medicare savings in the 1980s. Hospital benefits absorbed the largest share of all Medicare payments—nearly 68 percent in 1980 (Ways and Means 1991). And even though this share is now lower—44 percent in 1995—small changes still yield big savings simply because of the size of the pot. Moreover, the careful scrutiny of hospitals surrounding the introduction of PPS highlighted the strong Medicare profit margins enjoyed by hospitals, on average (ProPAC 1991). Policymakers reasoned that hospitals could afford to absorb further cuts and that the reforms in place allowed hospitals to change their behavior and avoid at least some of the negative consequences of reduced payments; they simply needed to become more efficient.

To some degree, attitudes about hospitals' abilities to absorb further broad cuts have changed. First, hospitals have not fared equally under Medicare (ProPAC 1991). As the controls have been tightened, some hospitals have become much more financially vulnerable. More hospitals each year are losing money on services to Medicare patients, with consequences that are very likely to spill over to Medicare beneficiaries and other patients as well. The discrepancies between hospitals that thrive under this system and those that face financial distress have been increasing over time. Ultimately, this disturbs more than just hospitals. Other insurers—fearing that Medicare hospital costs are being shifted to them and having their own reasons for seeking healthcare cost containment in the 1990s—are adding to the financial pressures on hospitals. Beneficiaries become concerned that the quality of care will suffer. Communities, which see hospitals as important employers, fear a shrinking wage base if hospitals are forced to close or severely economize.

Nonetheless, hospitals are still where the money is, and it is easier to portray them as bloated or inefficient than to make similar arguments for physicians or other small-scale providers. Individuals are often more sympathetic toward their own physicians.[3] Some investigators who monitor hospitals' response to PPS feel that hospitals have not moved far enough to introduce more efficient ways of providing services. Only further financial pressure would accomplish that. Thus, hospitals will still be a target of cost-containment efforts.

The PPS structure makes it relatively easy to make changes such as freezing or limiting the base payments for all hospitals. The annual market basket adjustment has often been reduced, and that could again offer a way to cut $10 billion or more over five years (Moon et al. 1995). And up until now certain special exemptions and protections have muted the PPS for some hospitals. This patchwork approach to protecting some categories of hospitals is coming under increasing scrutiny, however, as failing to eliminate inequities among hospitals under PPS.

Several approaches are possible to improve equity. First, PPS could be modified, perhaps as described in chapter 3, to better capture legitimate differences in costs across hospitals. Thus far, PPS has been unable to adjust for enough of the legitimate differences in costs to ensure that all hospitals receive reasonable levels of payment. One possible change in PPS would therefore be to reflect each hospital's historical costs in the payment base, rather than relying so much on national averages. Another adjustment would be to better reflect the needs of patients served by hospitals, such as adding indicators to diagnosis-related groups (DRGs) to capture severity of illness or other social factors that increase costs to hospitals of providing care. If such efforts are successful, then the burdens of further cuts would be more fairly distributed and targeted more fairly at hospital profits (called positive operating margins for nonprofit hospitals).

Another way to limit the inequities of cuts in hospital payments would be to focus change not on all hospitals but on certain categories of hospitals or specific hospital services. Teaching hospitals were given special treatment under the original PPS. But many of them now show relatively high Medicare margins (ProPAC 1995a). Since the initial adjustment giving teaching hospitals extra protection was set arbitrarily, these hospitals are a likely target for future cost-containment efforts. Even within this category of hospitals, however, some are currently struggling, so the problems of negative impacts on certain financially distresssed hospitals would not be totally avoided.

A strong argument can be made that medical education is not an appropriate cost burden for Medicare, since such payments are not just for Medicare beneficiaries' benefit—and should not, therefore, be financed by a payroll tax dedicated to funding hospital insurance for the elderly and disabled. Since direct and indirect medical education payments together represent about 8 percent of all Medicare spending on inpatient hospital care, shifting them outside the Medicare program would represent substantial savings to Medicare (although not to the federal budget as a whole) (CBO 1996a).

Disproportionate share payments constitute another specialized payment for hospitals, designed to protect hospitals that serve a high proportion of high-risk indigent patients. There is considerable evidence that this adjustment could be better targeted at hospitals that truly provide a great deal of such care (Moon et al. 1995). Such a change would generate savings both for Medicare and for the federal government as well. Finally, there is some evidence that Medicare payments for capital spending are now higher than needed to cover capital requirements. Reductions in this area may represent a reasonable policy change that would, again, save both Medicare and overall federal dollars (ProPAC 1995b).

While all these changes make sense separately, it is also important to consider their aggregate impact on specific hospitals. Teaching hospitals that also serve a disproportionate share of indigent patients may need special attention, for example. It is important to ensure that any combination of changes does not "pile on" the burden for particular hospitals. It is also important to understand that over time, there are likely to be fewer and fewer changes that can save money without threatening quality and access as Medicare and other payers continue to squeeze down on hospital operating margins.

Critics of hospital cost cutting, largely the hospital industry itself, also point out that the cuts since 1984 that have reduced the Medicare payment updates effectively serve to punish hospitals for achieving exactly what PPS sought to do: making profits by serving patients efficiently. When hospitals do well, the administration and Congress have felt confident in reducing the rate of increase in payments to hospitals. However, we have moved a long way in this direction already.

One other major area that will need reform in the very near future is hospital outpatient departments. This area is one in which Medicare continues to pay, at least in part, on the basis of incurred costs. However, cuts in this area have been ad hoc and have resulted in a crazy-quilt payment policy (Sulvetta 1992). Congress has already instructed the Health Care Financing Administration (HCFA) to devise a prospective payment strategy, but that effort has proceeded slowly; changes remain at the planning stage in 1996.

The rapid growth in this part of Medicare suggests that it is likely to serve as a major target for cost cutting in the future. Outpatient services by hospitals must increasingly compete with other settings. Ambulatory surgery centers normally receive facility payments below those offered to hospitals. Services provided in physicians' offices do not even have a separate facility payment. These alternative standards by which outpatient services can be judged suggest that payment levels can be brought down substantially. How to do so with a system of prospective payment that is simple, fair, and does not allow facilities to game the system to increase their payments over time is still an unresolved issue, however. To date, no scheme has been developed that meets all these goals.

Physicians

Physicians are the second largest source of Medicare payments after hospitals. But those who would target physicians for major cuts face a different problem. Since physicians are the point of contact of most beneficiaries with the healthcare system and the quality of care received depends enormously on these providers, policymakers have historically been reluctant to aggressively cut physician payments. First, there is fear that physicians may react by declining to treat Medicare patients. Second, the over 600,000 doctors in the United States represent a potentially formidable political presence. Third, patients, although anxious to see costs of care fall, are often reluctant to take on their own physicians.

Nonetheless, in 1992 after a period of transition, Medicare moved to a new fee schedule based on a relative value scale as described in chapter 3. Partially as a result of physician opposition, the initial fee schedule was intended to be budget neutral—that is, to generate no savings for the Medicare program. It did, however, reduce payments substantially for some specialties and treatment services as compared to more basic evaluation and management services.

Growth in physician services occurred at an average annual rate of 14.2 percent per year from 1980 to 1989 (Ways and Means 1991). Since the introduction of the new Medicare Fee Schedule (MFS), the rates have dropped substantially, in some years growing less than the rate of inflation in physician fees (SMI Trustees 1995). Future growth rates are expected to be higher, in the range of 7 to 8 percent (CBO 1996a), however, suggesting some room for further cuts.

Fears that physicians will stop treating Medicare patients have also receded, because those patients account for a substantial share of patient revenues. The American Medical Association (1991) reported that Medicare accounts for 26.7 percent of total revenues to physicians—although this proportion varies substantially across specialties. General practitioners and opthalmologists would likely find it difficult to turn away patients, whereas some other specialists such as orthopedists who now see few elderly patients are in a better position to do so. As Medicare's fee schedule is increasingly adopted by other payers, the threat of physician nonparticipation will fade even more.

Like the PPS system for hospitals, the MFS makes it relatively simple to cut payments by addressing the conversion factor which links the relative values of all services with dollars. Further, when specific services are identified that are "out of line," cuts in their relative values can be readily made. The largest impediment to such cuts, however, is that Medicare's payment levels are still below those of private fees—averaging only 68 percent of the private sector in 1995 (PPRC 1995). The relative decline in specialty and surgical fees makes the discrepancy in some areas even larger. Thus, it may be difficult to push Medicare physician fees even further until the private sector follows suit.

The Volume Performance Standard (VPS) provides another probable source for savings.[4] The VPS currently reflects a single national standard for two groups of services, surgery and nonsurgery. Although the original legislation left room for the VPS to be applied to more disaggregated groups to provide stronger cost-cutting incentives, current thinking leans toward collapsing the standard into a single category. Adjustments in the method of establishing the VPS level could then be used to create further Medicare savings (PPRC 1995). An alternative approach to achieve the same ends (Zuckerman and Holahan 1992) would base the VPS system on service *targets*. This would allow targeting of volume standards on services that are growing especially rapidly. This latter approach would emphasize making the adjustments reflect actual changes in behavior as compared to a more general feedback adjustor.

Also likely are changes designed to eliminate abuses. Legislative efforts to reduce the financial ties across providers that create incentives to undertake more tests and services have already been enacted. Efforts may also be made to check bills submitted by physicians, to ensure that they are not charging separately for services that are appropriately charged as a single service. These types of payment reviews are now used by private insurers and may well be adopted for Medicare. Fraud and abuse proposals, however, are often long on promises and short on expected savings. In the recent 1995 debate, for example, only about $4 billion out of the $226 billion would have actually come from all provisions to reduce fraud and abuse taken together (Moon 1996).

Other Changes in Provider Payments

Other areas of Medicare, which constitute a much smaller share of spending, are also likely to be targets for spending reductions. Outlays on home health services more than quintupled between 1987 and 1994, making this an area particularly ripe for policy change. The largest increases occurred in the average numbers of visits per user (Bishop and Skwara 1993). In 1995, over 60 percent of all visits were for beneficiaries with episodes of care lasting more than six months (Gage 1995). Further, since payments are still made on a cost basis, agencies are thought to have strong incentives to make as many visits as they can get away with. Changes in provider payments in this area are thus likely to focus not only on reducing payments per visit, but also on ways to reduce the number of visits received and provide stronger oversight of the use of this benefit.

Prospective payment systems will be difficult to develop in this area for two reasons. First, home health episodes vary substantially from short, post-hospital care to a more long-term benefit. Second, it may prove difficult to divide these episodes into discrete groups. Thus, an episode-based payment system may be infeasible, at least at present. Reductions in payment levels may help in the short run, while more sophisticated methods of profiling this benefit and a payment system that does not rely only on incurred costs are developed.

The skilled nursing benefit faces problems very similar to those found in home health services: lack of a prospective payment system and rapid growth in service (Moon et al. 1995). There is some indication that the use of ancillary services has been particularly important in driving up prices of skilled nursing care, offering another potential area for future reforms.

Recent budget proposals have also tackled payments to clinical laboratories, durable medical equipment suppliers, and hospice. None of these areas is very large as a share of Medicare spending, but as the search for savings in Medicare continues, almost no benefit area will be immune to cost-saving efforts. Billions of dollars are involved, however small the benefit, making it worthwhile to seek legislative changes in the rules for receipt of benefits, thus increasing the tendency to micromanage the Medicare benefit package. The risk is that such "reforms" end up complicating the program without always achieving the savings sought.

HMOs and Other Managed-Care Approaches

An increasingly common proposal has been to promote greater use of health maintenance organizations (HMOs) and other managed-care arrangements for Medicare beneficiaries, particularly as healthcare choices for younger families have increasingly moved in that direction. Moreover, such efforts could reduce the necessity for Medicare to oversee every aspect of the benefit package in order to contain costs. Under Medicare, the traditional approach has been to contract with provider groups to put them at risk for delivering care to enrollees. Under HMO contracts, for example, Medicare pays the HMO a flat rate per enrollee based on their characteristics (the adjusted average per capita cost [AAPCC, as defined in the appendix to this volume]).

After considerable growth in enrollee participation in HMOs in the mid-1980s, growth in the number of new participants slowed at the end of the decade, but then picked up dramatically in the early 1990s. By 1995, enrollment in Medicare's HMO program totaled 3.8 million, about two-thirds of whom are in risk programs. (Some beneficiaries sign up to participate in HMOs, but on a cost basis. These are usually beneficiaries who wish to remain with an HMO that served them when they were younger, but that does not have a risk-based contract with Medicare.) From 1993 to 1995, growth in HMOs averaged 17.7 percent annually, almost all in risk-based plans. Nonetheless, it will still take many years of growth as rapid as this for HMOs to dominate Medicare given the small initial base.

Moreover, we do not know how much has actually been saved to date from beneficiaries participating in HMOs. Medicare "saves" 5 percent on each HMO participant in the sense that the capitated rate is set at 95 percent of the expected expenditure level. However, there has been considerable controversy concerning whether these savings are in fact real. If, for example, the HMO can selectively attract enrollees who are healthier than average, or who have less propensity to use healthcare services, they may be skimming off enrollees who would never have cost Medicare the estimated expenditure level even if they remained in the regular fee-for-service part of Medicare. If that is the case, then Medicare would not actually be saving under this program. Indeed, the major studies conducted on HMOs in Medicare have found that there are actually higher costs associated with HMO enrollment after controlling for factors such as health status (Brown et al. 1993; and Langwell and Hadley 1989). If the best that can be achieved is a one-time 5 percent differential, after which expenditures rise at about the same rate as for all other enrollees in Medicare, this approach would not generate substantial savings over time, unless most beneficiaries enroll.[5] And unless the Medicare HMO payment rate (AAPCC) is substantially improved to capture beneficiary differences, savings will be suspect.

Medicare could try to further stimulate the market for managed care, but since Medicare wants to use this mechanism to save revenues, it makes no sense to do so by offering an increase in the AAPCC to HMOs. What other inducement mechanisms are possible? The program is now moving in the direction of encouraging less-formal HMO arrangements where beneficiaries can get services outside the network, a change that may further stimulate growth.

A go-slow approach to expanding HMO participation may be appropriate, however, until a better mechanism for paying plans on behalf of beneficiaries is developed. The rewards to HMOs for attracting healthy beneficiaries, particularly in areas of the country where the AAPCC is quite high, suggest that this is not a problem that will solve itself. In the interim, the Clinton administration has proposed savings from this part of the program by netting out the payments that are implicitly built into the AAPCC for the costs of medical education and disproportionate share subsidies that go to hospitals. Since the HMOs do not pass on these payments to hospitals, netting them out of the HMO payment seems reasonable. This would represent a reduction of about 5 percent, coincidentally an amount about equivalent to the last estimate of the overpayment of premiums due to the disproportionate number of healthy patients going into HMOs (Brown et al. 1993).

One note of encouragement is offered in a study by Welch (1991), who concluded that although the AAPCC formula has little cost-saving impact, HMOs have nonetheless served to decrease Medicare expenditures. Welch found that markets with large HMO shares lower the costs of care for everyone. If HMOs help change the norms for practice of medicine, they may be successful in lowering Medicare costs—even if they capture only part of the market.

Finally, it is very likely that expansions in some type of private plans will be an important part of Medicare's future. To make such efforts successful in both achieving federal savings and serving beneficiaries, it will be necessary to do more than just encourage greater enrollment. The major question is whether these changes will work within the current Medicare structure through modifications of the current HMO program, or whether more radical restructuring such as that discussed in the next chapter will occur.

Effectiveness Studies

Traditionally, new procedures or surgeries are introduced with few careful trials or tests of their effectiveness. And even if the procedures are effective for some, they are diffused to various groups or uses that may be inappropriate. Spurred by findings that some procedures are performed inappropriately in a substantial minority of cases, interest in analyzing effectiveness has grown. Studies by the RAND Corporation suggesting that procedures performed inappropriately both endanger lives and raise costs generated enthusiasm for what some have seen as a magic bullet: eliminate procedures performed inappropriately and achieve both improved quality and a reduction in healthcare costs (Brook et al. 1989). Accordingly, in the early 1990s, Congress and the Bush administration extended funding substantially in these areas. But ardor for such activity has waned, as efforts in this area also often identify underuse of some treatments and as critics question the appropriateness of government's role. Impatience with government testing for drug safety, for example, goes along with consumer impatience with constraints on their use of healthcare services. Whether in fashion or not, effectiveness research is an area where current investment could still pay dividends over time.

To fully utilize any findings in the search for cost savings, however, a number of additional steps would need to be taken. First, the results of effectiveness research must be widely disseminated. There is some encouraging evidence that when practitioners are aware that certain procedures are not desirable or effective, those procedures fall in volume. For example, as mentioned in chapter 4, evidence on Cesarean section for delivery of babies led to a decline in Cesarean births in the United States, but only after an education campaign (Myers and Gleicher 1988). This may be due to physicians' awareness and/or to the patients' awareness; in either case, the dissemination of information can change behavior.

Further, we need to increase our skepticism about the introduction of new treatments and new procedures without proper analysis of their effectiveness. Once treatments are in the mainstream of care, it becomes difficult to discourage their use. Again, economic incentives might be used to change behavior. Reimbursements under Medicare for new or experimental procedures could be lowered (or the cost share to patients raised) until their effectiveness had been determined. Technically, this is the rule. But it now applies only to high-visibility activities such as transplants. It should also apply to less dramatic procedures whose effectiveness has similarly not yet been proven. Currently, however, even when treatments have been shown to be ineffective, some Americans resist being barred from trying them. To entice doctors and patients to forgo accepted procedures just because they are not proven effective smacks of "rationing" in the American culture of doctor and patient choice, particularly when no alternative procedures are available. To forge a new public mandate would require a massive education campaign.

It is also important to note that constraints of these sorts need to be systemwide before they will be truly effective; we cannot rely on Medicare and Medicaid to discipline the whole healthcare system. Bringing more people under a public system is one approach. Short of that, the government could exert some systemwide control, perhaps by making the deductibility of insurance dependent upon insurers adopting practice guidelines.

True changes in attitudes will follow only if Americans are convinced that these controls represent good *health* policy rather than merely ways of holding down federal spending. Until we, as a society, begin to accept limits on what healthcare can accomplish, government standards and regulations will be unpopular and likely unsuccessful.

Cuts Directed at Beneficiaries

It is almost inevitable that some of the effort directed at cost containment will focus on requiring beneficiaries to pay more for their care. The rising well-being of the elderly as a group contributes to the perception that enrollees have the means to contribute. In addition, Medicare continues to be a very good deal for the elderly and disabled populations, paying substantially larger benefits than the size of workers' lifetime contributions. Of course, this could be an argument for higher tax contributions by workers as well as increased beneficiary contributions.

Throughout the 1980s, small increases in beneficiary liabilities constituted part of the strategy for reducing spending. Surprisingly, however, calls for greater beneficiary contributions were muted on both sides of the 1995 budget debate over Medicare.[6]

A small increase in the Part B deductible or premium of a few dollars per year only modestly expands the burden on individuals. But just $30 more per year from each enrollee would save the federal government over $1 billion. If the stakes are raised and the goal is to save $10 billion or more each year, it becomes more difficult to seek across-the-board increases from beneficiaries. Implicitly or explicitly, relating these payments to income becomes a more important option as part of any increase in enrollee liability. Without differentiating across individuals by ability to contribute, the feasible level of cost savings is restricted to what the lowest-income groups can reasonably afford to pay. (This issue is discussed further in an upcoming subsection.)

INCREASES IN COST SHARING AND PREMIUMS

Rather than just rearranging the cost sharing under Medicare, beneficiaries could be asked to pay more absolutely to help reduce federal spending on the program. This could be done through selective increases in cost sharing (recognizing the high levels already in place under Part A) or through a restructuring that would lower some required payments and raise others enough to result in net federal savings.

A reasonable cost-sharing package that simply increases enrollee contributions, for example, might raise the Part B deductible to $300 per year, and add a modest coinsurance premium of 10 percent of the average costs of a home health visit. Together these could raise about $5 billion per year in savings to Medicare (see table 6.2). These changes would place added burdens on beneficiaries, particularly the oldest and frailest who use home health and more physician visits, however.

Table 6.2 OPTIONS FOR RESTRUCTURING COST SHARING OF MEDICARE FOR ABOUT $5 BILLION IN FEDERAL SAVINGS IN 1996

| | Part A | | | | Part B | |
| | | Coinsurance | | | | |
Option	Hospital Deductible	Hospital	SNF	Home Health	Deductible	Monthly Premium
Current Law 1996	$736 for each spell of illness	$184 for days 61–90; $368 for days 91–150	$92 for days 21–100	None	$100	$42.50
1	Current law	Current law	Current law	10%	$300	Current law
2	$736 for no more than two stays/year	None	20% for all days	20%	$300	Current law
3	$736 first stay only	None	20% for all days	Current law	$300	$51

Source: Author's simulations using 1987 National Medical Expenditure Survey data, CBO 1996b, Federal Register 1995, and Health Care Financing Administration 1995.
Note: Table assumes changes are fully implemented in 1996.

To achieve about $5 billion in savings *and concurrently improve the cost-sharing structure*, more-dramatic increases in Part B deductibles and premiums would be required. The following set of changes represents a reasonable approach to improving the cost-sharing structure within the constraint of achieving overall savings. Hospital cost sharing could be limited to the payment of no more than two deductibles a year and the coinsurance for SNF care changed to 20 percent of the cost of all days in a stay. To fund this, the Part B deductible could be raised to $300 and a 20 percent coinsurance charge added for home health visits. The rapid rise in home health spending in recent years means that these changes would yield substantial additional savings. Alternatively, the deductible for Part A could be limited to only once per year. To cover this in the absence of any changes in the treatment of home health, the Part B premium would have to rise to 30 percent of costs (from its current 25 percent), or $51 per month in 1996.

These examples illustrate the inherent conflict between improving the cost-sharing structure and reaping net savings. As noted earlier, it is hard to go very far in restructuring without imposing extraordinary burdens on low-income beneficiaries or contemplating some form of income-related beneficiary contributions.

INCOME-RELATED BENEFICIARY CONTRIBUTIONS

As is abundantly clear from the earlier discussion of the Medicare Catastrophic Coverage Act (MCCA), any type of income-related cost sharing or premium runs a high risk of being attacked as contrary to the very intent of the Medicare program and undermining the strong public support for Medicare that continues even in the current climate of cynicism about the worth of government and government programs.

In fact, however, we have already moved to an income-related system with the Qualified Medicare Beneficiary (QMB) program, which survived repeal of the MCCA. The QMB program, managed through Medicaid, provides relief to very low-income Medicare beneficiaries by taking over their Medicare premium and cost-sharing liabilities.

The QMB program is limited to those with incomes under 100 percent of poverty and its companion program, the Specified Low Income Beneficiary program, pays the Part B premium for persons between 100 percent and 120 percent of poverty. A single person at 150 percent of the poverty guideline had an income of $11,610 in 1996. That person is devoting about 15 percent of his or her income on average to Medicare cost sharing and premiums—and a higher percentage for all healthcare spending—suggesting that relief further up the income scale is needed. Expanding the QMB program for persons up to 150 percent or 200 percent of poverty would help. But since a large share of the elderly have incomes in that range, such an improvement without offsetting increases in liability elsewhere would require a substantial contribution of new revenues. The QMB program is also unpopular with the states, because it competes with resources that might otherwise go to low-income families with children.[7]

An alternative would be to raise both Medicare cost sharing in general and the level of QMB protection. This would increase the amount by which cost sharing could rise without threatening beneficiary ability to pay. But in an era of projected cuts in Medicaid, new cost burdens are unlikely to be feasible for that program. There are two possible strategies. The first would be to raise the federal contribution for the QMB part of Medicaid close to 100 percent. This would keep the income-related part of Medicare in a separate program, preserving at least the claim that Medicare is not means tested. But it would obscure the full costs of covering the elderly and disabled. The second strategy would be to run the QMB program through Medicare. This would make the full costs of Medicare coverage apparent and the task of keeping the balance between the level of aggregate cost sharing and the resulting burdens on those with low incomes easier.

Another option would be to explicitly relate either Medicare cost sharing or the Part B premium to income. The challenge is to find a politically acceptable change that recognizes both the need for reducing federal outlays on Medicare and the limited ability of many seniors to take on ever-greater healthcare burdens.

What is the appropriate income level at which to begin increasing the premium? This is a difficult and ultimately subjective issue. Most proponents of an income-related premium advocate a starting point above $75,000 per year. But such premiums would affect very few people and hence would not raise much revenue.[8] An additional issue is what the maximum premiums should be, and that likely depends upon where the income threshold levels are set. Consider an example in which the premium is increased to a maximum of 75 percent of the costs of Part B for individuals with incomes above $80,000 and couples above $100,000 of income, and the phase-in for increasing the premium starts at $60,000 and $75,000 for singles and couples, respectively. For those with the highest incomes, the premium would triple, but revenues would increase by only about $2 billion (Moon and Mulvey 1995). The proposal contained in the Balanced Budget Act of 1995 (which was vetoed by President Clinton) would have increased the Part B premium to 100 percent of costs, eliminating the subsidy entirely for singles with incomes above $90,000 and couples with incomes over $150,000. This was projected to save $8.5 billion over seven years. If fully implemented in 1996, the savings would be less than $1 billion—about a 5 percent rise in premium revenues. To get more savings, the thresholds at which income testing starts would have to be lowered dramatically.

One of the biggest obstacles may be the practical problem of implementation. If an increased premium is assessed against only those with substantial incomes, it could be done through the income tax system with little further effort. But if a sliding scale is introduced that affects enrollees with modest incomes who do not now file an income tax return, the paperwork burdens on individuals would increase. Since the income tax is already an unpopular mechanism in general and also bears the baggage of the failure of the MCCA, it may be politically difficult. But creating a new administrative structure to oversee a new income-related premium would be cumbersome as well.[9]

It is interesting to note in this connection that we already have an income-related Part A premium through the financing side of the program. Legislation in 1993 required that, for higher income beneficiaries, 85 percent of Social Security benefits—rather than 50 percent—be included in income reported for income tax purposes. By including a higher share of these benefits in incomes, beneficiaries with incomes above $34,000 for singles and $44,000 for couples pay higher taxes than before and these taxes are dedicated to the Part A trust fund. In 1996, it is estimated that this provision will bring in $4 billion to the Part A trust fund (HI Trustees 1996). Thus, instead of adding a whole new administrative structure, at least in theory, this approach could be expanded to raise additional revenues in lieu of an income-related premium. That is, higher income beneficiaries could be required to report 100 percent of their benefits as income.[10]

Income-related cost sharing is even more complicated to introduce than income-related premiums. If the payment is collected by the providers, then enrollees may not only have to reveal their economic status to qualify for the program but make it known to their physicians and hospitals as well. One alternative is to cumulate cost-sharing liabilities, much as is now done with credit card charges, and have the government bill the individual directly. This relieves the provider and the beneficiary of paperwork and would keep the beneficiary's economic status confidential. (A proposal of this sort is discussed later in this chapter as an administrative improvement.)

This means, however, that the payment by the beneficiary is not made at point or time of service. Critics argue that payment after the fact eliminates the crucial deterrent effect of cost sharing, which is a major justification for relying on cost sharing; point-of-service payments relate the costs to the behavior. On the other hand, a quarterly statement detailing cost-sharing expenses might be sobering for many enrollees who currently lose track of how many physician visits and other services they have used.

If cost sharing is not to be assessed to change behavior, but only to require enrollees to pay more, it may make more sense to eliminate cost sharing and simply raise the average basic premium and add an income-related portion. The new premium could be set to fully offset the hospital deductible and coinsurance, and perhaps generate additional savings. Such savings could be part of the overall cost-containment effort or could be used to reduce the coinsurance on SNF care, for example. The advantage of this type of proposal is that it combines what should be a popular change (a benefit that simplifies and reduces point-of-service payments) with less popular change (an increased premium).

MODEST BENEFIT EXPANSIONS

Even if Medicare's finances are deemed so precarious as to preclude adding major new benefits, a number of small changes could enhance the well-being of enrollees without adding much to the fiscal burden. One of the important lessons of the MCCA, however, is to not oversell changes that make minor improvements but at some beneficiary cost. If, on balance, the goal is cost savings, it would be dangerous policy to suggest that a package of changes is for "Medicare enhancement," for example. Enrollees are likely to be as unforgiving as they were in 1988 if they believe they are being sold a bill of goods.

A major complaint by Medicare enrollees—and now a familiar refrain about the healthcare system in general—is the complexity of the program and the incomprehensible paperwork. Simplifications in the program's administration would be welcomed by beneficiaries. In addition, at a time when choice in the use of healthcare services is declining, greater flexibility in use of services may be important, particularly if it does not add to the costs. For example, expansion of the hospice program to make it a simpler and more readily available option could enhance patients' choices, at little additional cost. Finally, some modest expansions might be enacted such as adding more preventive services. More certainty about coverage for such services might result in better policy at moderate cost—and could be viewed as a simplification.[11] Each of these recommendations is discussed in turn.

Administrative Simplifications

Improved administration presents a broad area for policy change that runs the gamut from simpler, clearer explanations of benefits and reimbursement to major reform in streamlining payment of providers. It is not always a case of reducing bureaucracy and costs, as is often the rallying cry for administrative reform. Some areas need more attention, not less, adding modestly to the low administrative costs currently found in Medicare.

One simplification would be an improved enrollment card, much like a bank credit card, to be presented at the time of service. The Medicare card could work similarly to credit cards that are now scanned at the store, with information sent over the telephone wires to a central clearinghouse. For Medicare, this process could verify eligibility and record the charges. Medicare would pay the provider and the beneficiary would receive a monthly or quarterly bill. In a more sophisticated version, the bill could be sent to the enrollee only after the private supplemental insurance payment was also calculated. In the fall of 1991, Secretary of Health and Human Services Louis Sullivan met with private insurers to urge them to develop just such a billing system based on uniform reporting forms. But that effort has not come to fruition nearly five years later. Medicare could take the lead in implementing this change.

Such a streamlined system could reduce providers' hassle and paperwork enormously. Medicare could pay the full amount of the allowed charge and deal directly with the patient, rather than the provider having to seek payment from two sources. Just as improved administrative simplicity might secure some goodwill from enrollees in the face of higher cost sharing, providers might be less opposed to future cuts in their payments if some of their overhead were also reduced in this way. Medicare could also use the system to track and profile use of services on a patient-specific or provider-specific basis, an effort that is essential for better cost-containment activity in the future.

Opponents of such a system sound alarms at the centralized nature of the billing and information responsibilities that would be required of government, and important privacy issues are, indeed, involved. The system would also take cost sharing further away from the point of service, making it less of an immediate deterrent to service use. But such a step would also ensure that all Medicare enrollees have access to care, even if they do not have resources to pay at the time of service. If we move to a system of income-relating cost sharing, such a billing mechanism is particularly crucial, even though some additional administrative expenditures would be required—at least during the transition to this new system.

Billing service issues are important, but major improvement in communication with providers and beneficiaries requires more. Clearing up problems and getting simple answers to questions is still time-consuming and frustrating under Medicare's current structure. After years of effort to improve notices to beneficiaries regarding payment, they remain nearly unintelligible. Further, providers' problems increased with the decision to discontinue the toll-free line for physicians with reimbursement questions or complaints. The emphasis on scrutinizing and often disallowing claims as part of Medicare's cost-containment effort requires that the providers and patients who participate must be able to appeal or at least obtain the information necessary to interpret decisions that have been made. Educational efforts to help program participants understand the rules could result in better compliance. More, rather than less, effort needs to be devoted to these activities.

Finally, clearer instructions and oversight of carriers and intermediaries could improve the consistency of access to Medicare benfits. The discretion given these entities in their interpretation of different regulations results in very strict adherence to restrictions in some areas and much looser enforcement in other areas. Recent lawsuits concerning home health and SNF services have brought attention and some relief in this regard, but problems remain. These carriers and intermediaries also operate under very tight budget constraints, giving them few incentives to help providers and enrollees seeking clarification. Again, modest budget expansion is likely to improve services, which could pay dividends in compliance.

Hospice Care and the Last Year of Life

High-technology, expensive care for the terminally ill often makes little sense. Yet Medicare policy still treats such care as the "standard," and programs such as hospice care as less important and out of the mainstream. Elevating the status of hospice care would not be a large undertaking in terms of dollars, but an important symbolic one that could also yield major dividends in quality of life.

To qualify for reimbursement under the hospice benefit, patients must have a doctor certify that the patient has less than six months to live. The program then requires beneficiaries to forgo active treatments; in return, it covers more home health, some drugs, and other special services. But strict guidelines have discouraged many hospices from participating in Medicare. Such treatment makes hospices less available to patients and keeps them "stepchildren" of the Medicare program.

When added to Medicare, hospices were viewed as a benefit expansion, and the rules made restrictive enough to prevent them from adding to program costs. But such a rationale may prove penny-wise and pound-foolish. The view of hospices as a standard alternative to active medical care is one that advocates of deemphasizing high-tech care ought to espouse. But when Medicare restricts the role of hospices and limits their expansion, patients' attitudes are likely to reflect this vision. Also, as long as beneficiaries cannot participate until very late in their terminal illness, all other treatments are likely to have been exhausted and hospice may be an added service rather than an alternative.

The MCCA would have expanded hospice by eliminating the lifetime limit on the number of days covered. The Congressional Budget Office (1988) estimated the cost for that policy change at just $1 million per year. Since then, the program has been expanded, but further improvements are warranted.

Hospice care is not an "add-on" likely to be abused, or used prematurely; on the contrary, restrictive policies may dissuade patients from entering a hospice program at all, or lead them to delay entry if they fear that at some point benefits would be cut off if they are "unlucky" enough to be still alive at the end of the benefit period.

Eliminating the cost sharing now required under hospice care might also encourage further use. Even though such cost sharing is limited, it sends an important message. By treating hospice not only as a reasonable alternative but as one to be encouraged, attitudes about the use of life-prolonging technology might even be influenced, to the benefit of all. Further, if payments to facilities are too low or restrictive to encourage participation, even patients desiring such care will find it unavailable. In particular, current requirements that some services must be provided by unpaid volunteers may serve as a roadblock for expanding hospice programs. The original idea behind this requirement was to encourage community involvement. But it may be having the reverse effect of restricting access to hospice care.

Offering hospice or similar activities alongside other care in a hospital setting (a "quasi-hospice" approach) could be a good way of putting alternative treatments into the mainstream and altering attitudes of providers as well as patients. By providing such services in that more traditional setting, an individual would not be making such an absolute commitment to an alternative type of care. It might also enable earlier participation by those who wish alternative care. Patients in a "low-tech" wing might receive more nursing and social services in place of high technology, for example. Deductibles and coinsurance might even be waived for this type of hospital stay to encourage participation.

The bottom line is that if the patient's choice is to forgo treatment that would likely do little to meaningfully prolong life, the patient ought to share in the savings that could be generated. Positive economic incentives of this sort might undermine the prevailing attitude of "why not try the treatment since there is no cost to me." A careful analysis of the potential costs of alternative, low-tech care needs to be assessed against the possible savings from forgoing high technology. At a minimum, it makes little sense to restrict access to hospice care, and it may be cost saving to promote it.

Preventive Services

Preventive services is another area for possible modest expansion. The first steps were taken in this direction in 1988 with the MCCA, and the mammography benefit was resurrected in the Omnibus Budget Reconciliation Act of 1990 (OBRA). While most vaccinations are not covered, flu shots were added as a covered service in 1993. In theory, at least, other preventive services that the elderly and disabled populations might seek are not covered by Medicare. In practice, physicians and patients often engage in a "modest conspiracy" to obtain coverage by indicating that the physician is investigating a problem, in which case many tests and physician visits are thereby covered. Consequently, expanding coverage for preventive services is unlikely to offer as much of an expansion as it may seem at first. That means two desirable outcomes: costs would not rise as much, and all patients would be treated alike rather than restricting rewards to those willing to game the system.

Support for preventive services is frequently offered on the grounds of long-term cost savings to society by identifying and treating diseases at early stages. Many preventive services may well fit into that category. But preventive services for diseases whose incidence is very small would be very expensive relative to their benefits if applied as a routine screen. It may make more sense to cover only those with characteristics that make them more likely to be at risk. And in cases where there is a screen but no effective treatment we may be better off not even to screen. It is not at all clear that we should spend resources to identify diseases that we cannot effectively treat or for which there is no advantage in early detection.

For those who are otherwise healthy, preventive services may be the only ones received during a year. Such enrollees are unlikely to surpass even the current $100 Part B deductible. For this group, merely adding preventive services to the list of services eligible for reimbursement will not improve access. And raising the Part B deductible is particularly incompatible with the goal of increasing coverage of preventive services. One way around this might be to specifically exempt services from the deductible and allow them to be reimbursed at 80 percent of the fee schedule. A yearly cap could be placed on one physician visit and miscellaneous qualifying tests up to some dollar amount, for example. This option could substantially add to Medicare costs unless it was adopted in conjunction with a higher Part B deductible.

CONCLUSIONS

Ultimately, the modest reform alternatives discussed here are somewhat unsettling. The cost-containment strategies promise only small savings, not nearly enough to set the program on firm financial footing into the next century. Moreover, if any of the modest expansions were undertaken, cost-containment efforts might need to be undertaken just to "stay even." The suggested changes would improve the program in important ways, but they represent only a small step in reforming Medicare.

It is politically very tempting to stick with modest changes. The success and popularity of the Medicare program owes in no small measure to its stability. Wild swings in policy such as major restructuring efforts could undermine individuals' confidence in the program. And as was the case with MCCA, the losers may be more vocal than the winners if changes are designed to be relatively budget neutral overall. Finally, the implicit financial constraints on enacting even the very modest expansions discussed here dampen enthusiasm for needed changes.

Nonetheless, more substantive changes than those described here are needed. The options considered here do not generate sufficient savings to satisfy future needs for restricting the growth of Medicare, nor do they tackle some of the bigger gaps left in the program. Although the success of major changes would be greater in the context of systemwide healthcare reform, we should not wait for such broad reforms to consider options. At this point, even structural reforms to Medicare will have to be treated on their own merits. This is the task of the next two chapters.

Notes

1. For example, deductibles on conventional policies offered by employers of medium and larger firms averaged $257 per person in 1995 (KPMG 1995).

2. This would mean that Part B would need to become a mandatory program, however, and would necessitate a number of other adjustments. Mingling the various sources of revenue used to support Medicare—the dedicated payroll tax for Part A and general revenues and premiums for Part B—creates opportunities and challenges for financing.

3. This may be changing as well, however. A recent poll has shown that Americans are increasingly blaming physicians as well as others in the healthcare system (Henry J. Kaiser Foundation 1992).

4. As described in chapter 3, this part of the payment reform was a first attempt to control the rate of increase in Part B resulting from greater volume and intensity of services.

5. "One-time" savings may still have a substantial impact on spending over time. And if several are combined, the trend line in spending can at least appear to slow down.

6. For example, the Balanced Budget Act of 1995 (which failed to pass) would have modestly raised premiums for Part B and added a new income-related premium. But together these account for less than 20 percent of the total package.

7. Monies to support this program were supposed to come from savings to Medicaid from the MCCA expansions—but these were repealed in 1989.

8. Indeed, there are now proposals to begin income-relating (or even fully means-testing as will be described below) at much lower income thresholds. For example, Peter Peterson (1993) has proposed beginning the threshold cutoff for phasing out Medicare (and Social Security) eligibility at about $35,000 of income (with the actual amount tied to the national family median income). This proposal would affect many more people—and raise much greater revenues.

9. This way of income-relating the premium requires that the Social Security and Medicare systems be viewed in combination, likely to be a controversial issue for many supporters of Social Security.

10. This approach makes more sense if it is used to help fund a more substantial benefit increase such as long-term care.

11. All of these improvements could be undertaken without increasing overall spending on Medicare by more than $1 billion—and in some cases even less than that. In addition, improvements in Part A cost sharing could be undertaken with no offsetting increases elsewhere. This possibility was discussed earlier.

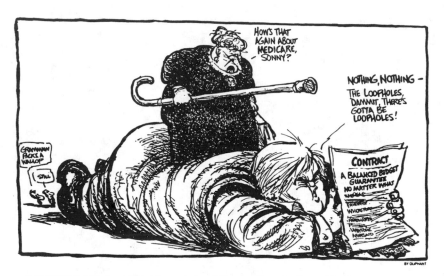

Chapter Seven

REDUCING THE COST OF MEDICARE

Any discussion of major options to shape the future of Medicare necessitates a delicate balancing of conflicting goals and strategies. The challenges facing Medicare in the wake of rapidly rising health-care costs and an increasing population of older persons signal the need for major changes in the program. Minor tinkering will be insufficient to hold down the costs of the program as we move closer to the 21st century.

By the same time the Part A trust fund is exhausted, shortly after the turn of the century, outlays under Medicare are projected to exceed income from payroll taxes by over $50 billion (HI Trustees 1996). At that point, the shortfall would represent about one-fourth of all Part A spending. Part B's funding is technically assured through general revenue support. But it too is growing at an alarming rate. To bring spending and revenue growth into balance will require more than minor changes in taxes and/or spending. Taxes could be increased to cover the projected shortfall in Part A, but that would require a substantial increase by the turn of the century and more thereafter. Medicare actuaries project that expenditures under Part A of the program, expressed as a percentage of taxable payroll, will total 4.6 percent in the year 2005, and rise to almost 5.1 percent by the year 2010 (HI Trustees 1996). If payroll taxes were increased to cover this shortfall through that period, they would have to be raised substantially from the 1.45 percent each currently levied on employers and employees to over 2 percent from each—a 40 percent increase in taxes. This does not include the general revenue increases that will be necessary under Part B, or the very high expenditures projected much later in the 21st century.

Resolving Medicare's overall solvency problem will require more dramatic changes than any discussed in the previous chapter. Among alternative strategies, major changes that affect beneficiaries directly need to be seriously debated. Both Republicans and Democrats have begun to test the waters with the suggestion that entitlements will "have" to be reined in. Whenever policymakers discuss cutting entitlements, Medicare is certain to be on the list, as illustrated by the debate over the fiscal 1996 budget in which the Republican Congress initially sought $226 billion in lower Medicare spending through 2002. And the Clinton administration proposed $97 billion in lower spending over that same period.

Major changes that would affect enrollees directly can be divided into three areas:

☐ Shifting risks onto beneficiaries;
☐ Reducing coverage of services; and
☐ Limiting eligibility.

SHIFTING RISKS

Options for shifting risk include (1) vouchers allowing beneficiaries to purchase the care of their choice and (2) a requirement that beneficiaries enroll in capitated plans such as health maintenance organizations (HMOs). Both options gain control over public spending on Medicare but do not necessarily protect beneficiary access to the same care they currently command. A voucher plan, for example, could give beneficiaries a set payment to purchase whatever type of health insurance they prefer—HMO coverage, some looser form of managed care, or traditional indemnity insurance—subject only to insurers meeting certain standards. Managed care options could require beneficiaries to enroll in HMOs or similar plans, the requirement being that the plans be certified by Medicare and overseen more directly—as is the case with the current HMO optional program.

Any option that increases beneficiary choice, however, faces the danger of risk segmentation—currently healthier beneficiaries systematically choosing different alternatives from currently less healthy beneficiaries.

Balancing Choice and Risk

One of the appealing aspects of restructuring from a beneficiary's perspective is the opportunity to choose among a variety of plans both in terms of the structure of the plan (i.e., fee for service versus health maintenance organizations) and also in terms of services covered. Beneficiaries can trade off higher premiums for lower cost sharing, for example. Some plans might emphasize long-term care or mental health benefits. Others might exclude such benefits as a means for lowering costs. The problem is that allowing choice concerning what services are covered is inevitably an invitation for plans to package services so as to attract healthy beneficiaries. Further, even if plans do not actively market to healthier groups, the beneficiaries themselves are likely to generate imbalances. For example, healthier beneficiaries who know they are less likely to use care in a given year are likely to choose plans with high deductibles and rebates—plans less attractive to those who know they will have substantial health expenses that year. Without adequate adjustments for payments to plans based on differences in risk, sicker beneficiaries would be severely disadvantaged.

Balancing between desirable choices and undesirable risk selection is not a problem with a simple solution, for Medicare or any other insurance program. The current method of paying managed care plans for Medicare patients is seriously flawed (see chapter 3), and we do not yet have the expertise to set risk adjustment factors to guarantee that insurers find older sicker patients as attractive as younger healthier patients.

Most restructuring proposals encourage development of optional private plans, often but not always featuring managed care, while keeping the standard Medicare fee-for-service approach as an option. The extreme variability in health outlays among beneficiaries, however, gives great leeway for plans to select relatively healthier beneficiaries for whom capitated rates exceed true costs. If sufficient protections to guard against risk selection are not in place, the standard Medicare option is likely to become a fallback Medicare program dominated by high-risk enrollees—persons with low incomes and/or health problems that make them unattractive to insurers. In this case, the costs of the Medicare fee-for-service program will skyrocket, not because of its inefficiencies but because of the high risk profile of beneficiaries who remain in that part of the program. In the longer run, this may not mean good news for private plans that participate in Medicare. If the very sick, low-income enrollees dominate the standard Medicare fee-for-service option, the premiums and cost-sharing requirements will become harder and harder to increase—with the inevitable result that Medicare payments to private plans will likely decline as well.

One way to minimize selection problems would be to make choosing a private plan mandatory. In this case the risk would shift fully to beneficiaries and/or private plans. Medicare would no longer be burdened with a high-cost fallback option. But that does not mean the selection problem would be eliminated. It simply means that some plans would face very high costs and high-risk patients would find it difficult to identify plans eager to take them.

A plausible outcome from such an approach is that out-of-pocket costs are pushed up substantially and many high-risk beneficiaries will move out of fee-for-service Medicare into managed care plans priced low enough to be affordable. These would likely be more restrictive than other, higher priced plans and might also be of lower quality. If the distinction begins to take place between high- and low-priced plans, Medicare may end up with a strongly divided program in which the goal of universal access to a defined benefit is lost.

Vouchers

Advocates of a private approach to financing healthcare for Medicare enrollees argue for a system of vouchers in which eligible persons would be allowed to choose their own healthcare plan from among an array of private options. For example, individuals might be able to opt for larger deductibles or coinsurance in return for coverage of other services such as drugs or long-term care. Since many Medicare enrollees now choose to supplement Medicare with private insurance, this approach would allow them to combine the voucher with their own funds and buy one comprehensive plan. No longer would they have to worry about coordinating coverage between Medicare and their private supplemental plan. One such approach which is increasingly being discussed would be a combined medical savings account (MSA)/catastrophic insurance arrangement.[1] Moreover, persons with employer-provided supplemental coverage could remain in the healthcare plans they had as employees. Other choices would allow for varying types of insurance, including managed care plans such as HMOs, preferred provider organizations (PPOs), or other hybrids.

The appeal of vouchers is that they allow government to control the rate of growth of program spending, effectively transferring the risk to the beneficiary or the provider. A Medicare voucher program would probably set the initial voucher price (the price of "choice") at 90 percent or 95 percent of the current level of Medicare spending per enrollee. The growth rate of the vouchers would then be set at some specified rate—the rate of growth of GDP, for example—regardless of the cost of private policies. This approach is often characterized as shifting Medicare from a "defined benefit" program to a "defined contribution" program. Limiting the growth rate of the voucher program in this way achieves major cumulative savings over time, and was essentially the approach taken in the 1995 congressional proposal for a voluntary voucher program within Medicare.

In the long run, federal savings from such an approach might be sufficient to keep within the bounds of payroll contributions, but only if this approach truly allows Medicare to permanently lower the growth rate in spending to about 5 percent per capita a year from the current rate of 8 percent. That means a reduction in the rate of growth of Medicare spending of more than one-third—an ambitious goal for any cost-containment program, public or private. Unless private insurers can find ways to achieve such massive reductions, the consequences of vouchers will be a shifting of the burden onto beneficiaries in the form of higher supplementary premiums. Advocates of vouchers argue that consumer opposition to paying higher prices would force insurers to hold down costs. Opponents claim that both consumers and insurers would lack the clout to achieve such cost controls.

How successful is the private sector likely to be in holding down cost growth? The task will not be easy: First, private insurers will almost surely have higher administrative overhead costs than does Medicare. Insurers will need to advertise and promote their plans. They will also face a smaller risk pool that may require them to make more conservative decisions regarding reserves and other protections against losses over time. These plans usually expect to return a profit to shareholders. All these factors cumulate and work against private companies performing better than Medicare unless other reforms occur. At least in the Medicare program, the government's track record at efficiently providing services is quite good, with overhead one-half to one-third that of the private market (CRS 1989).

On the other side of the ledger are the possibilities that private insurers may be able to devise new cost-containment schemes that will be more effective than either the private sector or Medicare have yet devised. They may be able to bargain for good prices and adapt to changing circumstances more readily than the public sector can. New types of HMOs or preferred provider organizations (PPOs) could even be developed. Finally, by combining coverage of those services Medicare now covers with other medical care such as preventive services, drugs, and long-term care, the private sector may be able to find better ways to package and deliver care than is currently the case in the public or private sector.

The experience of private insurers for supplemental coverage or coverage of younger populations gives little cause for optimism about how much more successful they can be than Medicare (Moon and Zuckerman 1995; ProPAC 1996). Healthcare costs in programs under the purview of private insurers grew as fast as or faster than Medicare costs in the last half of the 1980s. Moreover, private insurers have focused their competitive energies on policies that are at odds with the well-being of society as a whole. Insurers often hold down costs by selecting the groups they are willing to insure (the adverse selection problem discussed above in the context of choice within Medicare). Policies to exclude individuals with preexisting conditions or to discriminate against whole classes of individuals who may be more expensive to cover limit the insurers' risks, for example, but result in major gaps in coverage. Further, strategies of seeking discounts from providers for one group relative to others also saves costs for some at the expense of others. Larger groups with more clout implicitly penalize others. These activities do not hold down healthcare costs to society, but simply protect turf (Pepper Commission 1990). Moreover, Medicare already has held down payment rates, reducing the public/private contrast.

Regulation would be needed to require insurers to take all comers and to guard against problems of adverse selection. As noted above, achieving this goal may be difficult, particularly if some of the features that attract people to a voucher system are maintained. That is, if Medicare enrollees are free to supplement their vouchers to enhance coverage, insurers may find that those with the most to spend on certain types of supplemental coverage may be the best risks. The challenge would be to ensure that competition would truly be managed and not allowed to put beneficiaries at risk. Are proponents of competition willing to monitor it sufficiently to prevent these practices? A voucher system not only could allow the government to avoid making the tough calls, it also would give government a much lower stake in monitoring healthcare or contributing to efforts to restrain overall healthcare cost growth.

The most serious potential problem with vouchers is that the market would begin to divide beneficiaries in ways that put the most vulnerable beneficiaries—those in poor health and with modest incomes—at particular risk. If vouchers result in high cost, cadillac plans—or if other types of specialized plans (like medical savings accounts) skim off the healthier, wealthier beneficiaries—many Medicare enrollees who now have reasonable coverage for acute care costs but who are the less desirable risks would face much higher costs due to the market segmentation. A two-tier system of care could result, in which modest-income families are forced to choose less desirable plans.

Vouchers alone offer little in the way of guarantees for continued protection under Medicare. They are most appealing as a way to substantially cut the federal government's contributions to the plan indirectly through erosion of the comprehensiveness of coverage that the private sector offers rather than as stated policy. Leaving healthcare to the marketplace, especially in the absence of other reforms, would likely create more problems than solutions. Such an approach will only be successful if it is part of a systemwide move toward managed competition or at least combined with tough oversight and regulation. But this view runs contrary to what advocates of "privatization" are usually seeking.

Capitated Care Options

Rather than creating vouchers that put enrollees directly at risk, Medicare could move to a system of requiring managed-care arrangements. The program would still be operated and overseen by the federal government, so that the government could continue to share some of the risks. But enrollees could be required to operate within an HMO, an independent practice association (IPA), a PPO, or some other similar entity paid to offer healthcare on a per capita basis. All of these organizations seek to control costs by managing the overall level of care the patient receives, moving away from a system that pays on a per service basis where the more you use, the more the provider makes.

In a well-managed, high-quality, capitated system, the individual can receive much better continuity of care. Patient records and information can readily be shared within the organization, and services will be better coordinated. Physicians have no incentives to prescribe unnecessary tests or procedures, but they do have incentives to perform good diagnostic and preventive services, to reduce use of the big ticket items such as hospitalization. Private plans can not only provide closer oversight, they can also be more prescriptive than a national public program like Medicare. This means that, particularly in some areas like home health service use and hospital outpatient services, private plans could provide more controls on use of services than Medicare is currently doing. And while Medicare could certainly do better under its current structure, private plans may be better able to deal with providers who abuse the system by ordering too many tests or even deliberately defrauding the government. Private plans can simply exclude problematic providers or place restrictions on their behavior in ways that Medicare would find it hard to do. But, a caveat is important in this regard as well. Medicare's requirements for due process and other legal restrictions are not all bad. They help to guarantee access to all patients and providers to the system. It is important not to give up all such protections in enthusiasm over managing care.

In addition, managed care firms have not been anxious to move into the Medicare market. One size does not necessarily fit all in managed care, and firms that successfully manage care for younger persons may not find it easy to do well in this market. Older patients with multiple healthcare problems may need to see a specialist regularly, for example, when many managed care plans seek to limit such contacts. Other arrangements—perhaps agreements with specialists to be primary care gatekeepers, for example—may be more cost-effective for the Medicare population. It will take time for new entrants into this market to develop the expertise to deal effectively with this population.

Managed care systems mainly save costs by reducing use. This may reduce unnecessary care, but may also cut into important services because it may be easier to establish barriers to use of services than to carefully manage care on a case-by-case basis. This places a potentially substantial burden on consumers to be aggressive advocates for their own care. The barriers to care that HMOs and others establish to discourage overuse may be intimidating, particularly for the very old or frail. Further, the restrictions on choice implicit in such a system are viewed negatively by many.

Although HMOs generally have a reasonable track record in holding down costs, some critics argue that this is primarily a one-shot advantage. HMOs are able to achieve a one-time drop in use when people first enroll, but then the general trend in cost growth looks much like that for the fee-for-service sector (Newhouse 1985). If that is the case, savings would not be large enough to "solve" the financing problems of Part A, for example. And in the case of Medicare, the current payment structure effectively institutionalizes such an effect. It attempts to enforce a 5 percent differential with the fee-for-service side of Medicare but locks in a rate of growth which is the same as for fee for service. A major restructuring would also have to reform the payment mechanism, although for the reasons described above, a fixed rate is not necessarily appropriate either.

Medicare's experience with HMOs, as already noted, has certainly raised some concerns. Some HMOs have found it difficult to bring the elderly and disabled populations into their programs. Those that have attracted seniors have sometimes done so selectively, casting doubt on whether they are truly saving costs (Langwell and Hadley 1989). There have been some notable crises in which HMOs have suddenly dropped Medicare enrollees because of such financial difficulties (U.S. Government Accounting Office 1991a).

Determining a reasonable Medicare HMO payment per enrollee is inherently difficult. HMOs that select favorable risks have costs that are lower than the current AAPCC allocation. But HMOs that have not practiced risk selection have not always been able to cover Medicare patients adequately.

The promise of managed care and the pressures that will arise over time as the rest of the healthcare system moves in this direction make it imperative that Medicare improve its managed care efforts. But will such a shift lower the rate of growth sufficiently to achieve the stringent expenditure growth limits that some have in mind for the program? Or will stronger limits that effectively place both the insurer and the beneficiary at risk be required to meet those cost-containment goals? This is one of the major challenges likely to face Medicare for the foreseeable future.

REDUCING COVERAGE

If we cannot find ways to provide the same benefit package at substantially lower costs, we may turn instead to options for reducing covered services or the size of the subsidy under Medicare. It is important to keep in mind that this type of change simply shifts costs rather than changing the way in which care is organized.

Making Medicare the Insurer of Last Resort

One approach to reducing coverage would be for Medicare to become the insurer of last resort—limiting itself to protecting against truly catastrophic expenses. This would expand Medicare in some areas but result in a net reduction in coverage overall. Medicare now provides relatively good protection at the "front end" of health spending, requiring only a small physician deductible and no coinsurance for the early days of a hospital stay. But unlike most private insurance, it offers no limits on the total liability that beneficiaries may incur from hospital, physician, and other Medicare-covered services. Moreover, the coinsurance burdens increase for those with longer stays in the hospital or skilled nursing facilities—just the opposite of how most health insurance plans operate. Thus, in theory, Medicare does not operate like "insurance," which ideally seeks to spread the small probability of large losses across a population. Instead, it operates more like a prepayment system for routine expenses, covering, for example, physician office visits (above $100 per year) for over 80 percent of all beneficiaries.

A modest way to rebalance the program would be to eliminate hospital coinsurance and to increase the Part B deductible. But using restructuring to save the federal government $10 billion or more per year would require a much more dramatic change. This strategy was proposed by one of President Bush's healthcare advisors, but never turned into a formal proposal. One form these proposals have taken would trigger Medicare benefits only after an elderly or disabled person (or his or her private insurer) spends more than, say, $50,000 on care (essentially a lifetime deductible). Alternatively, individuals could be required to meet an annual deductible of, say, $3,000 before Medicare coverage began. After that, Medicare would step in and pay all healthcare expenses. Up to that point, individuals would likely buy private insurance as they do now, but at much higher premiums.

Under some versions of this plan, enrollees would also receive long-term care coverage—an option discussed in more detail below. But this approach could also be used just as a budget reduction plan. In that case the initial deductible might be set lower, but less would be added in "back-end" protection. Consider the case where the goal is to reduce federal outlays by $8 billion to $10 billion annually. One approach would be to eliminate all hospital coinsurance (as a way to improve protection at the back end), retain the Part A hospital deductible of $736 (to be assessed no more than once per year), raise the Part B deductible to $1,000, and offer some protection for those with lower incomes. This would save Medicare about $9 billion in 1996. Alternatively, the two deductibles could be combined into one deductible of $1,500. This would generate about the same level of annual savings.

These changes would aid the Medigap industry. But this approach would not lead to great improvements in the efficiency and simplicity of healthcare for the elderly and disabled populations. Private supplemental insurance has often been subject to abuse, and those who buy such coverage pay additional amounts for marketing and profits (U.S. Government Accounting Office 1991b). Private insurers also lack the market power to enforce cost controls on the healthcare system. This could place Medicare enrollees in the same disadvantageous position that younger persons in small group markets now face.

This type of change in Medicare could also lead to the perception by many beneficiaries that the program had been dismantled; it would operate more like reinsurance, backing up private-sector activities. If Medicare became "invisible" in this way, support for maintaining it could erode over time.

Substantially Increasing Medicare's Premium

A more direct approach would be to require enrollees to pay a larger share of costs of the basic benefit package. Currently under Medicare, an enrollee is required to pay a premium equal to about 25 percent of the costs of Part B.[2] But since this part of Medicare constitutes only 36 percent of total Medicare reimbursements, enrollees effectively pay a premium of 9.5 percent of the value of the total Medicare benefits they receive. If that premium contribution were raised to cover 20 percent of total benefits—a figure comparable to that often proposed in healthcare reform options as individuals' contributions—the current premium would need to be more than double its current level.[3] That is, in 1996, the premium would have to be $1,074 per year.

If applied to all beneficiaries, this would raise almost $21.5 billion in premium revenues. In practice, the net saving to the federal government would be less, since those below 120 percent of poverty would be eligible for protection under the Qualified Medicare Beneficiary (QMB) program. Net federal savings would likely be about $19 billion after accounting for the increased Medicaid burdens.[4]

However, although this 20 percent premium would be consistent with employer-subsidized plans. Medicare benefits are also less comprehensive than those offered to younger families and many older Americans must pay all or a substantial share of the costs of supplemental Medigap premiums. Since premiums for standard plans tend to average about $800 to $900, Medicare beneficiaries in total are paying premiums that are substantially higher as a proportion of coverage costs than those paid by many younger families.

In addition, although modest increases in premium contributions, as discussed in the last chapter, could be absorbed by many Medicare beneficiaries without great difficulty, increasing reliance on this mechanism to "solve" a large portion of the financing problem for Medicare would necessitate an income-related approach, if extraordinary cost burdens on moderate-income beneficiaries are to be avoided. A single individual with an income at 150 percent of the poverty line (about $11,600 in annual income in 1996) would be paying 9.3 percent of his or her income for the premium alone. Even at 200 percent of poverty, the premium would still command 6.9 percent of a beneficiary's income. When other costs of care from both Medicare cost sharing and noncovered services are added to this burden, most moderate-income Medicare enrollees would be *routinely* spending 30 percent or more of their incomes on healthcare.

The challenge is to find a politically acceptable change that recognizes both the need for reducing federal outlays on Medicare and the limited ability of many seniors to take on ever-greater healthcare burdens. If the limits where income-related burdens begin are set high, they will raise few new revenues. But to get substantial increases in revenues means higher premiums on middle-income families, which will be much less popular politically. Many of the 1994 reform proposals advocated an income-related premium, suggesting that the fears from the negative reaction to the Medicare Catastrophic legislation have waned over time and that premium changes are likely to come in some form in the near future. All those proposals, however, would have affected only a small number of beneficiaries, since they would not begin to take effect until annual incomes reached at least $75,000. More dramatic moves to reduce Medicare's spending would require the income cutoff for such premiums to be lowered considerably.

The traditional way to think about an income-related premium is for one or a series of increases to be added at the top of the income distribution. But an alternative would be to expand the QMB program and then phase it out gradually as income levels rise, in concert with a general overall increase in the Part B premium.[5] These constitute very different philosophical approaches. The focus of the traditional income-related approach is on distinguishing between moderate- and high-income beneficiaries. An expanded QMB approach concentrates on protecting low-income beneficiaries from increases. A combination of the two approaches is also possible.

Most of the traditional income-related proposals that have been offered add a new premium on top of the existing Part B premium. It is usually phased in for individuals or couples above a particular level of income, reaching a maximum for all persons above some higher income cutoff. Such a strategy allows the top premium to be much higher than the level feasible under a flat premium increase. For example, the proposal contained in the Clinton health reform bill of 1993 would have added a new 75 percent premium to be phased in beginning with single persons with incomes over $90,000 and for couples with incomes over $115,000. Other proposals go as far as requiring beneficiaries to pay the full actuarial costs of Part B for those in the top tier.

What is the appropriate point to begin increasing the premium? This question has no "right" answer. Most proponents of an income-related premium advocate that the rise in premiums not begin until people have incomes above at least $75,000 per year. Since such premiums would affect very few people, they would not raise large amounts of revenue. Opponents of income relating fear that this is just the beginning, however, and that the thresholds would be lowered over time.[6] How high should the premiums be raised? That depends upon where the threshold levels are set. If the thresholds are very high (say, $60,000 or $75,000 in income for a couple), then it is feasible to raise the share paid by beneficiaries to a higher level than if the thresholds affect those with more moderate incomes.

To illustrate the revenue impact of several different alternatives, consider two different approaches, each with a range of income cutoffs (table 7.1). The first approach would income relate the premiums while retaining the existing QMB program. The second would expand the QMB program to 150 percent of the poverty guidelines and move it to Medicare.[7] Two income cutoff levels are relevant, as already noted. The first represents the point at which the premium begins to rise with income. The second is the point where the maximum is reached. This set of examples assumes that the premium rises steadily between the two income levels. Distinctions between singles and couples yield four sets of numbers.

Several conclusions emerge from table 7.1 First, it is the increase in the bottom tier premium that boosts savings the most. The option in which the bottom tier stays at 25 percent raises the smallest amount of revenue, even when the top percentage is 75 percent (compare options 1 and 3). Second, at the high end of the income distribution, lowering the top tier income cutoff substantially does not increase savings by very much. Compare, for example, options 2 and 3, in which the income phase-in drops by $30,000 from $90,000 to $60,000 of income for singles. Savings only increase by $600 million. This suggests that setting the income level at which the maximum premium is charged at a relatively high income level may reap political gains without reducing savings very much. Third, in the lower part of the income range, dropping the phase-in and maximum income cutoffs increases savings dramatically (compare options 4 and 5). Finally, increasing the QMB protection (on the assumption that participation increases and there is full federal funding) reduces the savings that would otherwise accrue.

Taxing the Value of Medicare Benefits

Another alternative for shifting the cost burden onto beneficiaries in a way that is related to income would be to treat Medicare benefits— all or in part—as income subject to the federal personal income tax.

Table 71 ESTIMATED REVENUE INCREASES AS A SHARE OF CURRENT PART B PREMIUM FROM INCOME-RELATED OPTIONS, 1996

Option	Premium Tiers as Percentage of Part B Costs	Top Tier Income Phase-In for Singles/Couples ($)	Top Tier Maximum (Singles/Couples) ($)	Revenue Increase in Billions	
				Continuation of Existing QMB Program	Expanded QMB Program
Current (1996) law	25%	—	—	0	0
1	25% & 75%	60,000/75,000	80,000/100,000	$2.0	$ – 1.0
2	30% & 75%	90,000/105,000	115,000/130,000	4.8	1.1
3	30% & 60%	60,000/75,000	80,000/100,000	5.1	1.5
4	30% & 75%	60,000/75,000	80,000/100,000	5.7	2.1
5	30% & 60%	25,000/30,000	32,000/45,000	10.7	7.0

Source: Author's estimates using March 1993 Current Population Survey.

If, for example, half of the average value of benefits were added to the incomes of elderly and disabled persons, these benefits would be subject to tax rates that would vary according to other income received. This would naturally result in a progressive tax on Medicare benefits. This is analogous to taxing Social Security, although it is more complicated because these benefits are received "in-kind" and are not traditionally viewed as income by the beneficiaries.

Not only would such a tax raise program revenue, but it would make beneficiaries more acutely aware of the "value" of Medicare benefits and their rate of growth over time. If a portion of benefits were taxed, but only for those whose incomes are above some threshold, the extra burden would be restricted to high-income beneficiaries.[8] This could preserve universal eligibility for Medicare without a means test and still ensure that high-income elderly pay more.

Taxing benefits would be a substantial change in policy—one that would add considerably to the complexity of the program while raising relatively small amounts for Medicare. Critics of this approach also argue that it is unfair to tax some in-kind benefits and not others. And consistent treatment of health benefits would require taxation of benefits offered by private employers—another controversial policy.

How much would such taxation yield? Taxes as a percentage of benefits total 2 percent under Social Security's current taxing scheme, which has a threshold of $25,000 for singles and $32,000 for couples. If the same scheme had been applied to Medicare in 1992, it would have raised between $2 billion and $2.5 billion, compared to $6.2 billion for Social Security (Ways and Means 1992). Lowering the threshold would increase the yield—but would reduce the progressivity of the tax. The Congressional Budget Office (1994) projected savings from a range of lower thresholds for 1994 between $4.7 billion and $10 billion. The same CBO study pointed out that progressivity could be increased, for example, by exempting some entitlements or establishing a threshold of income before taxation begins (similar to what now happens under Social Security). If all entitlements were subject to taxation, 60 percent of the elderly would be affected and benefits would effectively fall by about 11 percent. This would raise approximately $20 billion in 1996.

LIMITING ELIGIBILITY

The third cost-control element under the control of the federal government—in addition to shifting risk and reducing coverage—is who participates in the program. Reducing the number of beneficiaries could also generate substantial savings. But how to do this?

Increasing the Age of Eligibility

The initial age of eligibility for Medicare could be increased as one way to limit eligibility.[9] One of the justifications for such a change— aside from the primary one of saving the system money—is that as the life expectancy of the population has increased, the normal age of retirement should also increase. Since Medicare was introduced in 1966, life expectancy for persons ages 65 and older has increased by a little more than two years (U.S. Bureau of the Census 1995c). As people live longer, they now receive Medicare benefits for a greater share of their lifetimes. Increasing the age of eligibility could bring this proportion back to the level anticipated in 1965. In fact, this approach has already been adopted for retirement benefits under Social Security. The Social Security amendments of 1983 established a schedule by which the age of eligibility for full Social Security cash benefits would increase over time from age 65 to age 67 by the year 2027.

For Medicare, the transition would need to be more rapid than this, since the financial crisis for Medicare will come sooner than that for Social Security. Age eligibility could be increased by two months every year for a period of time. Alternatively, the phase-in could begin more slowly at first and then accelerate.

Raising the age of eligibility for Medicare would create problems. First, moving too rapidly creates problems for people near retirement age or who have recently retired, and who have made their financial plans based on outdated assumptions about the availability of Medicare coverage. Second, and more fundamentally, not all Americans are equally healthy at age 65. Although life expectancy is increasing over time, the health of persons in each age range has not shown similar improvement (Poterba and Summers 1985). And whereas some Americans remain in the labor force or have generous retiree benefits at age 65, others struggle to make it to that age to qualify for Medicare. Many older persons who retire earlier or are moderately disabled at, say, age 62 or 63, are in poor health and are poor candidates for purchasing insurance on their own.

To make this option less burdensome on those individuals, Medicare could change in other ways, allowing for at least partial eligibility for all those ages 65 and above. (This option could be analogous to early retirement benefits under Social Security, which are now available at age 62—an alternative that will be retained after the full retirement age rises, albeit with greater reductions in benefits.) For example, full eligibility might be retained at age 65, but a higher premium (either fully recouping the actuarial costs or a portion of them) could be charged to enrollees between the ages of 65 and 67. In that way, Medicare would be available for those who must retire early. If this is also combined with some low-income protections and phased in slowly, the objections of critics could be effectively addressed.

The disadvantage of this more modest approach is that it limits and postpones savings to the federal government. Further, while many persons age 65 through 68 would be more able to afford higher premiums than are the very old, this is a rather imperfect way to differentiate among individuals on the basis of ability to pay. Of persons aged 65 and older, 46.6 percent have per capita incomes less than $10,000 per year. Of those aged 65 to 68, 37.6 percent also have incomes below $10,000 (U.S. Bureau of the Census 1995d), still a substantial group.

Age Rationing

Another option that would effectively restrict eligibility by age is the proposition by Daniel Callahan (1987) that beyond a certain age, only palliative care should be offered. This means no heroic efforts to sustain life for persons above an age limit such as 75 or 80. Proposals for age rationing of healthcare stem from the economic arguments that we are spending too much on medical services and that something must be done beyond the usual tools of cost containment. Age is viewed as a proxy for determining who is not a good candidate for certain types of services.

This approach is not likely to be enacted in the U.S. context, and there are good reasons to argue against it. First, the problem of excessive use of medical care by the elderly is overstated. Moreover, the evidence does not support holding the elderly totally responsible for spending decisions. Adopting a cure such as age rationing may prove to be worse than the disease.

Take a look at who is responsible for the high costs of healthcare. For all types of care and for individuals of all age groups, use of healthcare services has risen dramatically over the last 20 years, although healthcare spending has grown faster per capita for the elderly than for other age groups (Meyer and Moon 1988). Studies of the growth of spending generally cite a number of contributing factors:

healthcare price inflation, the aging of the population, technology, and a general increase in the number of services. Inappropriate use of health services and the impact of technology on spending in healthcare are the most logical areas for focusing attention. It has become fashionable to associate such expenditures with the last year of life. Are we devoting an increasing share of our health resources in vain attempts to forestall death—often through new technology? Certainly, few statistics sound as compelling as Lubitz and Prihoda's (1984) widely quoted finding that 28 percent of Medicare spending is concentrated on the 5 percent of enrollees in their last year of life. This finding and other similar ones are cited by those who believe that a key to controlling healthcare spending will be to limit spending on the very old.

But is such rationing a magic bullet that would reduce healthcare spending in the United States? A careful look at the data suggest that the answer is not nearly so simple. First, if technology is being used ever increasingly in futile cases involving the very old, the share of resources devoted to healthcare in the last year of life should be rising. The evidence, however, does not support these claims. Lubitz and Riley (1993), updating the 1984 Lubitz and Prihoda study, found that between 1976 and 1990 (a period of enormous cost growth in healthcare), there was little change in the share of Medicare resources going to those in the last year of life.

Further disaggregation of Medicare data reinforces this analysis. If we look first at expenditures by age in Medicare (figure 7.1), the familiar pattern of more spending on the very old emerges, seemingly supporting claims of disproportionate spending on this age group in hopes of sustaining their lives just a bit. But the data show exactly the opposite pattern by age for persons in *their last year of life* (figure 7.2). In this case, we spend considerably more on the 65- to 69-year-olds than on those age 85 and older. Effectively more is spent on younger Medicare beneficiaries who are more likely to recover—a result consistent with reasonable healthcare policy. Since life expectancy at age 65 is now over 17 years (U.S. Bureau of the Census 1995c), spending on the younger old is not necessarily just cheating death for a few months but, rather, treating patients with many useful years left.

These findings suggest several things. First, physicians do not always know that death is imminent when making healthcare spending decisions. And since people often die after being ill or requiring medical treatment, it is only natural to see extraordinary spending on those who die (as well as on those who survive a major illness). The more appropriate issue is whether we disproportionately spend on

Figure 7.1 MEDICARE SPENDING BY ALL ELDERLY BY AGE, 1986

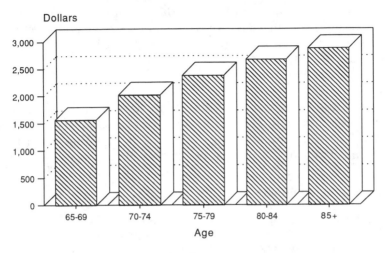

Source: Health Care Financing Administration (1990).

Figure 7.2 MEDICARE SPENDING BY DECEDENTS BY AGE, 1985

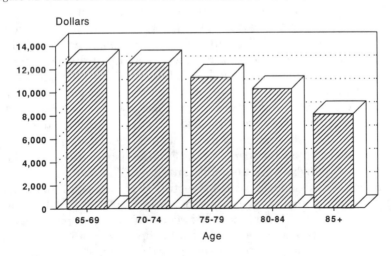

Source: Lubitz (1990).

those with no chance of survival and whether that contributes substantially to the problem of the growth in healthcare spending. The evidence does not support this conclusion. There is a drop-off in spending on the very old compared to the young in their last year of life, suggesting that, at least on average, decisions are being made to resist heavy acute-care expenditures on the very old who are terminally ill.

Given these caveats, it is difficult to imagine how to design a reasonable age-based rationing policy that would save substantial dollars for the federal government. Age rationing is certainly not a magic bullet; indeed, it would likely prove to be a quagmire.

Means Testing Medicare

The ultimate extension of income-related cost sharing is to make Medicare a means-tested program—available only to persons whose resources are below some specified limit. Higher-income elderly and disabled persons could be offered the option of either buying into the system at a nonsubsidized rate (such as is now done for persons over age 65 who are not eligible for Social Security benefits) or of being precluded from participation altogether. The former is likely to be the more cost-effective approach, since there might be savings to participants from the economies of scale and low administrative costs of more rather than fewer Medicare enrollees, even if no formal federal subsidy is involved.

The main justification for moving in the direction of means testing is budgetary savings. Advocates of a means-tested approach also argue that Medicare is not a sufficiently progressive program, since everyone eligible has access to the same benefits. In this connection, it should be noted that although the financing for Medicare is not progressive, the combination of benefits and taxes does result in a program where higher-income beneficiaries pay a greater share of the costs (through payroll taxes assessed over their working lives). For example, contributions from a salaried individual making $100,000 per year total $2,900, compared to the $20,000 per year worker whose combined employee-employer contribution will be $580.

A major argument against means testing Medicare is political. Such a change would likely undermine the strong support that has traditionally gone to Medicare precisely because it is a universal program. It would constitute a major shift in philosophy from a universal to a "welfare"-based program. As discussed in chapter 2, the drafters of the legislation were very cognizant of what they were doing when they stipulated that the program would include all of the elderly. They knew the political value of a program that would be viewed as a "middle class" entitlement.

A major practical concern is where to set the cutoff for eliminating eligibility. At what income is an elderly person capable of footing the bill for the full costs of Medicare? Consider 1995 levels of spending. In this case, the average Medicare subsidy was $4,300 and the enrollee's liability was $1,261 (Federal Register 1995). Together this total of $5,561 would consume a substantial share of the income of most enrollees. For the elderly, Medicare out-of-pocket costs average about half of the total out-of-pocket liability they have each year. Other uncovered expenses such as prescription drugs account for a substantial additional portion of their incomes. Thus, per capita liabilities just for acute care would be about $7,000 in 1995. In that same year, the average elderly person had an income of about $11,000.

If policy were set so that the average expenditures on healthcare should not total more than 20 percent of an individual's income, the cutoff for eligibility for Medicare would be set at $35,000. If the figure used instead were 15 percent, the income cutoff would rise to $45,000. These levels would mean that very few elderly persons would be excluded from Medicare. In 1993, only 8 percent of the elderly had per capita incomes in excess of $35,000 and only 3.7 percent had incomes in excess of $50,000 (U.S. Bureau of the Census 1992a).[10] Eliminating eligibility for those with incomes above $35,000 would save the federal government an estimated $13 billion—about the same amount as a number of less dramatic options. To avoid the problem of an enormous "notch" where people just above an income cutoff receive nothing and people just below receive the full subsidy, a phaseout would be needed. For example, the subsidy could be reduced beginning with those whose incomes were $35,000 or more, and then eliminated at, say, $50,000. The subsequent federal savings would be substantially lower—totaling only an estimated $9 billion.

CONCLUSIONS

To achieve savings in excess of 10 percent of Medicare spending in any given year, several of the preceding options might need to be enacted. For the most part, each of the options described would save no more than $10 billion if fully implemented (in 1996 dollars). With any political compromise, the amount of savings would be less. Cost-savings estimates of the "moderate" versions of various options discussed in this chapter are summarized in table 7.2.[11]

To fully means test Medicare is the least appealing approach in table 7.2. It would fundamentally alter the nature of the program without achieving more savings than other less draconian alternatives. The same savings, with less angst, could be achieved by increasing—and income relating—the Part B premium. The examples in table 7.2 indicate the effects of varying stringency in income cutoffs, and show that means testing could raise less than other options. Income relating the premium or taxing the value of the benefit reduces subsidies gradually, rather than abruptly as under a means-testing option.

Table 7.2 OPTIONS FOR ACHIEVING MEDICARE SAVINGS

General Approach	Specifics	Approximate 1996 Savings ($ billions)
Increasing Medicare premium	Raise basic Part B premium to 30 percent and begin increasing to 60 percent for those with incomes above $25,000 (singles) and $32,000 (couples).	11
Restructuring to make Medicare more catastrophic	Eliminate Part A coinsurance and limit deductible to one per year. Raise Part B deductible to $1,000. Increase QMB protection.	9
Limiting Medicare through vouchers or HMOs	Pay 90 percent of AAPCC toward costs of healthcare premiums. Beneficiaries would enroll in private plans and be at risk if costs grow over time. Assume includes one-third of all beneficiaries (instant phase-in).	6
Means testing eligibility for Medicare	Restrict eligibility to persons with incomes below $50,000 (or charge premiums of 100 percent of cost). Phase out eligibility with higher premiums on those with incomes over $35,000.	9
Taxing the average value of Medicare benefits	Tax one-half of Medicare benefits for persons with incomes over $25,000 (and couples over $32,000) by adding to income subject to personal income tax; at $34,000 and $44,000, raise share to 85% of HI and 75% of SMI.	7
Increasing the age of eligibility for Medicare	Raise eligibility by one month per year until eligibility age reaches 67, starting in 2000.	—[a]

a. Savings would grow faster than other options over time, but would not go into effect immediately.

Raising the age of full eligibility for Medicare may constitute a reasonable approach, but it needs to be phased in over time. It is thus more appropriate for the longer run and is a less-than-satisfying option for those who wish to see large savings right away. Increasing the age of eligibility could be combined effectively with premium increases to achieve greater beneficiary-based savings. But a higher age of eligibility would also need to be combined with other reforms in private insurance or allowing individuals to buy into Medicare to protect those at younger ages who would lose eligibility for Medicare. It is also important to note that most of these savings to the federal government translate directly into higher costs for beneficiaries. These proposals, then, are not so much cost containment as cost shifting.

One major option that has received considerable attention in the last several years is to shift much of Medicare to private plans via a voluntary voucher approach. But as shown in table 7.2, this would not necessarily save a very large amount, at least initially. The dilemma is that under a voluntary system, plans must attract beneficiaries. Plans will only want to do so if they believe they can offer attractive options and still do well financially—goals that require that Medicare pay a reasonable premium on behalf of beneficiaries who sign up with private plans. But higher Medicare payment levels imply lower savings to the program. Table 7.2 assumes both that payments are reduced to 90 percent of the AAPCC and that one-third of all beneficiaries sign up—the proportion likely to enroll after seven years, according to CBO estimates of the 1995 congressional plan. A mandatory voucher, on the other hand, may simply become a regressive way to shift costs to beneficiaries.

Just as there are advocates of doing less under Medicare, many supporters of the program would like to see it expanded, perhaps funded by some of the reductions described here. Although reductions in spending are much more likely in the next few years, proposals for expansion are the subject of the next chapter.

Notes

1. This option, which was a prominent feature of the congressional plan offered in 1995, would allow beneficiaries to use their Medicare subsidy to buy a high deductible catastrophic plan and place any remaining subsidy in a medical savings account that the beneficiary could then use to pay expenses below the deductible. The biggest concern from this and other related approaches centers on the question of whether the

Medicare payment to individuals can be adequately adjusted for risk. That is, if this option attracts mainly healthy individuals and if Medicare were to make a payment to the insurance company setting up this arrangement that reflected the overall risk profile of Medicare beneficiaries, the federal government would lose money compared with the status quo.

2. In 1995 that percentage had risen to 31.5 percent because for several years the actual dollar value of the premium was established in legislation, and forecasts of Part B costs overestimated how high the premium would have to be to equal 25 percent.

3. If such a policy were adopted, it would make sense to combine the two parts of Medicare and require participation in Part B.

4. Some of the increased Medicaid burdens would be borne by the states, unless the Qualified Medicare Beneficiary (QMB) program were to be shifted to Medicare. In that case, only about $15 billion would be saved. This option is discussed in chapter 8.

5. At present the QMB program creates a "notch" in which persons with incomes $1 below the cutoff are eligible for full protection while those with incomes $1 above that cutoff receive no help. A gradual phase-out of this benefit would thus improve its equity.

6. Indeed, there are now proposals to begin income relating (or even fully means testing as will be described below) at much lower income thresholds. For example, Peter Peterson (1993) has proposed beginning the threshold cutoff for phasing out Medicare (and Social Security) eligibility at $35,000 of income (with the actual amount tied to the national family median income). This proposal would affect many more people— and raise much greater revenues in consequence.

7. Since the QMB program is now part of Medicaid, and because many states were traditionally reluctant to add those to their programs, some of the low participation in the QMB program would likely be helped simply by putting it in the Medicare program. In that case, we assume that participation would rise to 70 percent of all eligibles. This change also means that the federal government would have to bear costs now the responsibility of states.

8. Again, this is comparable to how Social Security is now treated in the tax code. In that case, the thresholds are $25,000 for single individuals and $32,000 for couples. These thresholds limit substantially the number of elderly and disabled persons who are taxed on their Social Security benefits.

9. This option was proposed in the Senate version of the budget debate of 1995, which sought to balance the budget over seven years. The increase would have begun in the year 2000.

10. Options to eliminate Medicare for the very well off are effectively symbolic gestures that save little, at least initially. For example, just 2 percent of households with the head over age 65 have incomes above $100,000 (U.S. Bureau of the Census 1991a).

11. The only option missing is that of age rationing, which would not raise sufficient funds to justify such a controversial cost-containment approach.

Chapter Eight

EXPANDING MEDICARE

Unmet needs for services now excluded by Medicare can only be accommodated by substantial increases in spending. In the current environment, where the costs of healthcare are very high and 38 million persons are covered by Medicare, even relatively minor expansions of the program implicitly become major options for change because of their budgetary implications. To slow the growth in Medicare and at the same time absorb the costs of an additional $8 billion or $10 billion annually in expansions would be a formidable task. Even during the national health reform debate in 1993–94, expansions proposed for Medicare were very modest.

Nonetheless, proponents of expanding Medicare can make a strong case that there are gaps that could be filled in to better serve beneficiaries. But even the most ardent supporters of such change generally temper their options with modifications that result in less than fully comprehensive expansions—limiting the types of new benefits or eligible enrollees, or requiring offsetting changes elsewhere in the program. These options, which cover both acute- and long-term care concerns, are discussed here.

IMPROVING ACUTE CARE

Despite concerns about the cost of Medicare and the fiscal crisis ahead for Part A, expanding Medicare's coverage and eligibility is still being discussed. For many, improved protections for those with low incomes or high health expenditures top the list of concerns. The possibility of adding coverage of prescription drugs was discussed at the time of Medicare's passage, was included in the Medicare Catastrophic Coverage Act of 1988 (MCCA), and remains on the wish list of groups such as the AARP. Further, there are many advocates for lowering the eligible age to 62, even as much of the policy debate is focusing on raising the age of eligibility from 65 to 67. Some also seek to expand eligibility to disabled persons immediately upon becoming disabled. They must now wait 29 months after onset of the disability to receive Medicare.

Moving an Expanded QMB Program to Medicare

The Qualified Medicare Beneficiary (QMB) program was established as part of the Medicaid program in the MCCA and was one of the few elements retained after repeal. Its goal was to extend protection for low-income Medicare enrollees against the costs of Medicare's cost-sharing and premium liabilities. Medicaid has traditionally reached only about half of the elderly poor. The MCCA required that everyone up to the poverty line receive at least the fill-in protection for Medicare-covered services.[1] And the related Specified Low Income Medicare Beneficiary (SLMB) program provides protection for those between 100 and 120 percent of the poverty level against the cost of Medicare premiums. Funding for states to meet these new responsibilities was to come from a shifting of costs from traditional Medicaid beneficiaries to Medicare as a result of the expanded coverage under the MCCA. But when the Medicare portions of the MCCA were repealed, state Medicaid programs were left with increased responsibilities but no offsetting decrease in demands elsewhere.

Particularly during the recession of the early 1990s, states argued that the new QMB burdens were forcing their Medicaid programs to underserve other important groups such as mothers and children. Perhaps because of the resistance of states, the QMB program got off to a slow start, with low enrollments by eligible Medicare beneficiaries. Since public policy now seems to be in the direction of greater state flexibility, the QMB and SLMB programs may be at risk in the future if left to states' discretion.

One option for addressing the pressures on Medicaid from the QMB program and for extending relief somewhat higher up the income scale would be to shift it formally into the Medicare program. This could provide important relief to Medicaid, making it more difficult for Medicare to shift future burdens of healthcare for the elderly and disabled onto that program.

Medicaid would mainly provide supplemental acute-care benefits that Medicare does not cover. It would reduce fragmentation and confusion by collecting all the public responsibility for acute care for the elderly and disabled under the Medicare program. And it would have one major additional advantage. It could increase the use of the QMB and SLMB benefits by those eligible for it. Current participation areas are 63 percent for QMB and 10 percent for SLMB. These rates are low. Making the programs part of Medicare (a popular universal program without stigma) would facilitate efforts to increase participation, which would increase the fairness of the Medicare program—treating equals equally. If QMB and SLMB participation increased to 70 percent and 20 percent, respectively, in 1996, the cost of this improvement in equity would be about $6 billion.

At current levels of out-of-pocket burdens on Medicare beneficiaries, protection might also need to be set higher than 120 percent of poverty. This becomes more and more important as other changes to increase premiums and cost sharing are debated. For example, if the Part B premium were increased, the SLMB protection level might be expanded to 150 percent of the poverty guidelines, easing the burdens of an across-the-board rise in premiums. Those eligible might be required to pay the premium on a sliding scale so as to eliminate the "notch" effect that comes when one additional dollar of income moves a person from full eligibility to ineligibility for any protection.

A practical issue that would arise in moving the QMB program into Medicare is eligibility determination. Medicaid now has a mechanism for determining eligibility in terms of income and asset holdings. Should Medicare continue to contract with Medicaid for this service (and risk keeping participation low), or should it establish a new mechanism within Medicare for testing eligibility, which would be expensive? How much additional administrative cost can be justified depends in part upon whether an income-related premium for individuals above the Medicaid cutoff is added to Medicare as well. In that case, the payoff to adding new administrative structures to Medicare might justify testing of income for QMBs and SLMBs as well.

Finally, less dramatic reforms might include increasing the federal government's share of the costs of the QMB and SLMB programs, thus reducing state objections to this part of Medicaid. One way to do this would be to charge states only a part (say, half) of the premium costs for buy-ins for eligible Medicare beneficiaries.

Adding Stop-Loss Protection

One of the areas of greatest concern to health policy professionals in assessing the quality of health insurance is whether it offers good stop-loss protection—that is, the guarantee that above a certain threshold, the individual should not have to continue to pay out of pocket for covered services. This is one of Medicare's greatest weaknesses; there is no limit on the amount of cost sharing that beneficiaries are theoretically liable to pay.

Ironically, however, this is not how many beneficiaries view the coverage problem. Traditionally, Medicare enrollees have been more concerned about choosing supplemental policies on the basis of first-dollar rather than last-dollar coverage. Further, objections to the MCCA were that the benefits were not the ones most desired or valued by enrollees. Nonetheless, adding good stop-loss protection to Medicare would be an important improvement in the program's fundamental insurance function. Finally, many beneficiaries already implicitly have such protection once their supplemental insurance or Medicaid is taken into account. And QMB protections offer stop loss for eligible persons.

A proposal to limit liability on the Part A side was described in chapter 6 in the context of modest program changes, combined with an option to finance it. But stop-loss protection was not discussed there because of the high costs of adding such protection. The combination of limiting Part A liability for hospital costs as discussed in chapter 6 and capping out-of-pocket liability for Part B services at $1,700 was costed out for 1992 in the context of the MCCA debate at $5.7 billion (Congressional Budget Office 1988).[2]

The net increase in spending would be moderated today, however, because the QMB program now provides stop loss for those with the lowest incomes—about 10 percent to 12 percent of Medicare enrollees—reducing the costs of the program by a similar proportion. After accounting for increased spending on Medicare and more beneficiaries overall, a stop loss of $5,000 would cost Medicare about $9 billion in 1996. Even at this level of expense, the protections are not very generous for low- and moderate-income beneficiaries who are above the QMB protection levels, but who would still find out-of-pocket expenses of up to $5,000 catastrophic. A $5,000 cutoff is still low enough to be expensive to provide but high enough to still be a substantial burden for those with modest incomes.

Expanding Eligibility for Medicare

The two groups most closely related to existing Medicare beneficiaries are early retirees between the ages of 62 and 65 and newly disabled individuals who have qualified for Social Security (after a 5-month waiting period) but then must wait an additional 24 months to receive Medicare. Both these groups receive Social Security, and in that sense are recognized as needing public support. And both may have special healthcare needs that render private insurance either expensive or unavailable at any cost, particularly given the failure to pass private insurance reforms that would allow individuals guaranteed access to affordable insurance coverage.

PERSONS AGED 62 TO 65

Most Americans under the age of 65 receive their health insurance through the workplace. But workers aged 62 to 64 are less likely to have such coverage, and those who retire before age 65 are at additional risk of being uninsured. Anecdotally at least, it appears that employers are beginning to scale back their retiree health benefits (Foster-Higgins 1995). Many early retirees and their families live on modest incomes and may not receive retirement benefits from former employers. In 1988, 10.2 percent of all persons aged 62 to 64 had no insurance from any source, and another 16.9 percent relied on private, nonemployer coverage.[3] Women are disproportionately likely to have no insurance (10.9 percent) or to have only nonemployer coverage (20.1 percent) (Moon 1991a).

This age group may get some relief from legislation passed in 1985 requiring employers to allow employees who leave the firm or dependents who have a change in status (such as a divorce or being widowed) the option of buying into the group health plan (referred to as "COBRA protections"). But there are limits on how long persons can keep such coverage, ranging from 18 to 36 months. And more important, even when available, these benefits may be too expensive for departing workers, who must pay the full costs of the coverage. Survey data indicate the average monthly premium for a conventional group plan was $185 for individuals and $454 for families in 1994 (KPMG 1994).

Privately purchased nongroup coverage is usually more expensive than group plans. People aged 62 to 65 have substantially higher health expenditures on average than younger age groups, and the cost of individually purchased policies normally varies by age. Thus, if nongroup insurance is experience rated, costs to early retirees for individual coverage could be $300 to $400 per month. Affordability issues can thus extend to families with incomes well above the official poverty thresholds. And individual nongroup insurance is not just expensive, it also often excludes coverage for preexisting conditions for a period of time (typically a year, but in some cases indefinitely).

Several groups of Americans in their early 60s are particularly at risk.[4] A majority of early retirees have little choice in the timing of retirement and receive neither pensions nor good health benefits.

These individuals may have faced a period of unemployment before deciding to take reduced Social Security benefits. They may have had only sporadic periods of employment or have worked in jobs without insurance. For early retirees, Social Security benefits will be less than if they had postponed retirement. They are also likely to lack private pension coverage, further limiting their retirement incomes. They may also be in poor health. A recent study of retirees aged 51 to 61 found that many of them had health problems (Loprest 1995). Such problems can make continuing in their current jobs untenable. They can also make it difficult to purchase insurance at any price.

DISABLED PERSONS

Persons who qualify for Social Security disability must still wait for 24 months to obtain eligibility for Medicare. During that waiting period, the lucky ones may have private coverage or be eligible for Medicaid. COBRA protections, for example, are guaranteed not to run out during the waiting period. But for those who do not have access to COBRA or other group insurance, finding insurers who will cover a totally and permanently disabled person may be difficult indeed. Almost by definition, such individuals will have important preexisting conditions that may preclude them from buying coverage or from getting insurance to cover their problems. Experience from Medicare indicates that such individuals have very high levels of health expenditures.

Further, disabled individuals tend to have low incomes; to qualify for Social Security they must be unable to work, so unless other family members work, Social Security benefits may be the main source of income for many disabled persons. Average monthly Social Security benefits for disabled workers were $662 in 1994 (Social Security Administration 1995). Consequently, elimination of the waiting period for Medicare would relieve these individuals of an important burden.

EXPANDING COVERAGE TO THESE GROUPS

Medicare is potentially a logical source of coverage for disabled and older Americans who are without employer-based coverage. Early retirees, spouses of Social Security beneficiaries, and recently disabled persons have much in common with current Medicare beneficiaries. Health expenditures for 60- to 64-year-olds look much like those for 65- to 69-year-olds. And newly disabled persons would likely have health expenses comparable to long-term disabled persons. Thus, the needs of these groups are quite similar to those of current benefici-aries. Moreover, the rationale for coverage is much the same: these are people outside the mainstream of employer-covered insurance who will ultimately receive Medicare coverage. It makes sense to create a reasonable transition to Medicare benefits for them.

How should the premium price be set for such buy-ins? At one extreme individuals could be required to pay the full actuarial value of the coverage. In 1996 the full actuarial premium for Parts A and B is $459 per month. This option has two disadvantages. The first is that it would be affordable by, and therefore help, relatively few people. The second disadvantage is that it would create problems of adverse selection. Those with the option of COBRA coverage are likely to choose that option because the actuarial cost of many employee groups is lower than that of the group that would be eligible for the buy-in. The group without a COBRA alternative would have individ-ual private coverage as their only alternative to the Medicare buy-in. Because of Medicare's low administrative cost, the Medicare buy-in, even at full cost, would be cheaper for them. But the non-COBRA group is less healthy than average for their age group, resulting in adverse selection for the Medicare buy-in group. This adverse selec-tion would raise the actuarial cost of the Medicare buy-in, further reducing the attractiveness of that option for the healthy with other alternatives, and further aggravating the adverse selection problem.

It thus makes sense to offer at least enough subsidy to limit the adverse selection problem and ensure that the public option will be as affordable as many employers' group premiums. A limited subsidy starting at age 62 would be consistent with the structure of Social Security. Federal savings from raising the age of full eligibility might be used to help finance this liberalization for those under age 65 so the full range of subsidized coverage could extend up to, say, age 67.

Many of the poorest members of this group will continue to find insurance unaffordable, however, if the subsidy is only enough to make the Medicare buy-in competitive with COBRA coverage. And most disabled persons would not be able to afford coverage unless it were generously subsidized. Thus, many members of the group most at risk would still be uninsured.

But a very generous subsidy creates other problems. If it induces those who now have private insurance to turn instead to Medicare, increased coverage for the group that needs help will come at the expense of also subsidizing many who now have reasonable coverage. Employers who now offer coverage may decline to do so in the future if the Medicare option is available. Relatively well-off early retirees may prefer subsidized Medicare coverage. The result would be Medicare substituting for private coverage rather than expanding coverage to groups that would otherwise be uninsured.

A combination of subsidies would help this problem. Moderate subsidies could eliminate any bias in costs from adverse risks—by pricing premiums assuming the costs for the full pool of persons in the age category, for example. Income-related subsidies could then be added to help protect those who could not otherwise afford insurance.

Adding a Prescription Drug Benefit to Medicare

The major uncovered items on the acute-care side are prescription drugs. Except when administered to patients in a hospital, nursing home or, to a limited degree, hospice program, regardless of how essential the drugs are to a patient's course of treatment, Medicare does not pay. This is the one area where Medicare coverage remains substantially less comprehensive than the standard policies available for most Americans through their employers.

Many, but not all, elderly persons who have Medigap coverage are able to get private supplemental insurance for drugs. But the best drug benefits are available to the relatively well-off elderly who have retiree coverage that brings their insurance up to the level of what was available when they were working (NCHSR 1989). Drug coverage purchased directly by the elderly is inherently expensive, since the elderly are disproportionately large consumers of drugs. Moreover, prescription drug coverage is sought more than proportionately by those who know they need it, creating additional pressures on price from adverse selection.

The only relief is from special drug programs that some states offer for low-income elderly persons that fill some of the coverage gaps. These are in addition to the drug benefits provided through the regular Medicaid program (all but two states offer drugs under Medicaid) (Soumerai and Ross-Degnan 1990).

Lack of coverage for prescription drugs can actually raise the costs of Medicare-covered services. Failing to fill their prescriptions altogether or cutting back on the amount they take make beneficiaries' conditions worse and lead to more acute problems that require hospitalization and additional medical expenses. One recent study on a Medicaid program that limited prescriptions for enrollees found that such a policy resulted in additional admissions to long-term care facilities and ultimately much higher costs than if all the necessary drugs had been available (Soumerai et al. 1991). In that case, not covering drugs clearly constituted a penny-wise but pound-foolish policy.

The problem, of course, is that adding prescription drug coverage to Medicare would substantially raise overall direct costs to the federal government. Out-of-pocket spending on drugs is estimated to have averaged $246 per elderly Medicare beneficiary in 1994 (Moon and Mulvey 1995). And those with drug coverage in their Medigap policies are likely to pay a substantial amount in additional premiums for that coverage. Many individuals now are able to pay for their prescriptions, so any savings in avoiding complications from not taking drugs will certainly not be sufficient to counteract the cost of making that coverage available to everyone. The prescription drug program that would have been available under the MCCA was estimated to cost $2.2 billion in 1991, despite a $600 deductible and 50 percent coinsurance (Congressional Budget Office 1989a). That number was projected to double in 1992, to $4.4 billion (when the program would be fully phased in with a 40 percent coinsurance and a $652 deductible). Reducing the deductible or coinsurance and updating these costs to 1996 would further increase the estimate.

ADDING LONG-TERM CARE

The hardships that the costs of long-term care impose on individuals and their families can be staggering. It is hardly surprising, then, that the strongest candidate for expansion in the eyes of Medicare beneficiaries is long-term care.[5]

Medicare began as an acute-care program and as yet covers very few of the long-term care needs of the population over age 65. Periodically, groups concerned about the elderly and disabled populations note the inadequacies of Medicaid, the primary public source of support for long-term care, and call for Medicare to offer a broader benefits package in this area. However, proposals to expand long-term care coverage through Medicare are very expensive. If coverage were to be provided under the same terms as current acute-care coverage—universal coverage only partially paid for by the recipients themselves—costs might range as high as $80 billion. Thus, a full-fledged long-term care plan would require a sizable new financing mechanism.

At present, long-term care is funded mainly by Medicaid, individuals, and their families. Medicaid provides mostly nursing home coverage, with eligibility limited to individuals who have spent down their income and assets to very low levels.[6] It essentially offers protection after the catastrophe has already occurred. Middle-income people benefit from the program, but only once they have already devoted most of their resources to paying for care. Medicaid has been characterized as insurance where the deductible is your lifetime savings and the coinsurance is your annual income. For most American families, this represents a very bleak option.

It also makes little sense for individuals to rely only on their savings to meet long-term care needs because these needs are not predictable. Most people will not require such care, but for those who do it can be very expensive. In a sense, this is the perfect "insurable" event, in which the risks ought to be shared across a large group. But the private sector has been slow to develop such insurance policies, despite a well-demonstrated need.

Why can't individuals simply seek long-term care insurance products through the private market? Insurers are understandably cautious about marketing products where the liabilities will not be known for many years. This conservativeness, combined with the costs of marketing and selling to a largely nongroup market, may make the price too high for many persons aged 65 and over.

Further, private insurers often offer coverage only to individuals in good health at the time of enrollment. In addition to current disability, individuals with hypertension, arthritis, any history of heart disease, diabetes, or recent hospitalizations may be screened out. As yet, there is little evidence that such factors are actually good indicators of later need for long-term care, but, nonetheless, individuals with such medical histories are unlikely to be able to purchase individual long-term care insurance policies.

Short of a comprehensive social insurance approach (discussed in the next section), a range of options are possible that would limit overall public costs. Only some services might be covered, such as home health, while leaving nursing home coverage under the Medicaid program. Alternatively, coverage could be broad but limited to only lower-income Medicare enrollees. Or, long-term care services could be added in exchange for reduced benefits on the acute-care side. Over a longer time frame, long-term care services could be added as an insurance benefit with only modestly subsidized premiums— although this approach is less compatible than the others with the structure underlying the rest of Medicare. Finally, any or all of these programs could be made optional.

Comprehensive Long-Term Care Coverage

In the aggregate, the financial resources required to provide long-term care services to all those in need sobers even the most sympathetic legislators. In an era of fiscal austerity and concern over reducing the federal budget deficit, enacting a public, comprehensive long-term care system is almost always viewed as a policy goal beyond our collective means. Nevertheless, there is considerable public support, backed by reasonable arguments, to move in that direction. National polls indicate that the American public strongly favors a universal, public-sector approach to solving the problem of long-term care (Moon 1989). In addition, even strong advocates of private "solutions" to the problem recognize that there will always be gaps and unmet needs. A comprehensive approach, which by definition is universal, is seen by many as offering the best possibility of achieving: 1) equitable treatment for those in need, 2) control over administrative costs, and 3) the orderly development of a reasonable delivery system.

Society as a whole is now bearing much of the cost of long-term care, but in ways that place enormous burdens on a few. Some of these are very visible costs: the $44 billion that Medicaid spent on long-term care in 1993, and the even larger amount that individuals and families pay. There are also invisible costs in the sacrifices that families make and in the unmet needs that result in suffering and reduced quality of life.

A universal program could also help ensure access to quality care. Leaving the current system intact or encouraging private insurance will result in two distinct worlds of long-term care services and delivery. Already many providers concentrate on the "private" market, discriminating against Medicaid patients. Medicaid, as a welfare program, provides low payments in many areas, and providers know that private-pay patients will bring in more revenues and greater profits. Naturally, private-pay patients are preferred to Medicaid patients, often resulting in the seemingly contradictory findings of empty beds and waiting lists under Medicaid. Although a two-class system of care is, to some extent, inevitable, having most people in the public program would help safeguard the quality of the publicly funded care.

A comprehensive program could also be efficient. Social Security and Medicare have both proven to be very effective in holding down administrative costs. For example, Medicare is able to return about $0.97 in benefits for every $1 of financing. A public system would clearly benefit from having the largest possible risk pool over which to spread both risks and costs. Moreover, a public program like Medicare has no marketing or advertising expenses. Finally, the delivery system for any long-term care program will be an essential element in determining whether needs are met at reasonable cost. A single system for reimbursing providers offers opportunities to mold an as-yet-undeveloped delivery system and to use prudent purchasing to hold down costs of care.

A system relying on private insurers plus Medicaid would continue the patchwork system that has developed over time in the long-term care area. And form is likely to follow reimbursement. If private insurance continues to focus on nursing homes, for example, home care will continue to lag. If the emphasis in private insurance is on more rather than less formal home care (as seems likely for purposes of accountability), we may have a more medically oriented long-term care system than anyone believes is desirable.

A universal system would undeniably result in increased costs of long-term care. Those who now postpone or avoid getting services because of the fear of being on welfare or the inability to qualify would become eligible. In addition, expansion of covered services into community and home-based settings would encourage users who wish to avoid institutionalization at all costs. Although such expansion may be politically difficult, it should not be decried as bad simply because costs would rise. Indeed, meeting unmet needs should be a goal of an expanded system, and some increase in expenditures on nursing home and home and community services should be welcomed. Nonetheless, as stated earlier, the issue of cost is compelling. It is hard to advocate spending an additional $60 billion to $80 billion under a program that is already facing severe financial constraints.

Other arguments against moving to a universal public long-term care system also exist. Many proponents of other Medicare expansion options advocate expanding the acute-care side before turning to long-term care. Moreover, since the elderly are increasingly viewed as a "privileged" group, expanding benefits to this population before solving other problems may be politically untenable. Indeed, many critics of expanded long-term care protection contend that it would serve mainly to protect the assets of the upper middle class and preserve inheritances. If so, this would not be the most efficient or desirable use of public dollars.

Moving to a national universal system could also lead to inflexibility. Services now vary dramatically from location to location in the United States; what works well in Buffalo, New York, may not be easily transported to a small town in Arizona. Long-term care likely does not need to be as standardized as the acute-care system to be efficient and of high quality. Thus, fitting everything into one mold may not be the best approach, and could lead to added costs over time.

An Income-Related Benefit

An alternative to a comprehensive approach, in long-term care as well as other areas, is to develop an income-tested benefit. Such an approach would cost substantially less, depending, of course, on what cutoffs are set. If the limit allows for protections that would be meaningful to many middle-class elderly or disabled families, even maintaining a spend-down type of program may be acceptable. For example, if asset protection levels were set at $30,000 and $60,000 for singles and couples, respectively, nearly 60 percent of the elderly would not have to spend down any assets before becoming eligible (Moon 1993). Once eligible, the individual or couple could be assessed a substantial copayment of perhaps 40 percent or 50 percent of the costs of their care if their incomes are above a certain level. This type of income relating would leave most individuals eligible for at least partial benefits. The other approach is to totally exclude those with incomes above a certain level, but such a direct move away from universal coverage would almost certainly be politically unpopular in the Medicare context.

The major barrier to an income-related long-term care benefit added to Medicare is the inconsistency of fully protecting the assets of a rich older woman facing gall bladder surgery (acute care) but not those of her neighbor who must be sent to a nursing home to recuperate from a broken hip (long-term care). The two beneficiaries will perceive the coverage difference as inequitable, since to them the same issues are involved in the two events. Thus, if the long-term care benefit is to be highly income related, in the absence of similar changes on the acute-care side it may make more sense to create a separate program for long-term care, or to continue to use Medicaid for the purpose.

Limited Expansion of Medicare Benefits for Long-Term Care

Perhaps the simplest small-scale expansion of Medicare to cover long-term care would extend the existing skilled nursing facility (SNF) and home health benefits to a broader range of needs for elderly and disabled people. These two programs are now restricted to ensure that they do not offer true long-term care benefits. SNF coverage requires that the patient need either skilled nursing care or rehabilitation services. In addition, it is limited by a three-day prior hospitalization requirement and a very high coinsurance payment after 20 days that effectively makes the benefit worth much less after that time. Home health is also a skilled benefit, limited to certain services. It does not have the same limits on days of coverage as SNF, however, and has grown more rapidly over time. And in the last few years, critics contend it has begun to serve long-term care needs.

Several simple changes could substantially expand the help that Medicare offers to enrollees with chronic care needs. First, the SNF changes that were part of the MCCA could be reinstated. Eliminating the prior hospitalization requirement, expanding coverage to 150 days per year (with perhaps a lifetime limit of 300 or 450 days), and reducing substantially (or eliminating) the coinsurance would likely extend coverage to many more persons. Early analysis of the impact of those changes suggested an immediate response by providers and beneficiaries (Liu and Kenney 1991).[7] This initial response to MCCA has also carried over, keeping use of services relatively high for SNF care.

These benefits would aid those who will have short nursing home stays and eventually return to the community. For such individuals, the burdens of having to spend down to become eligible for Medicaid are particularly harmful, since they will return to the community with fewer resources to meet other needs. But not all beneficiaries needing long-term care, even for short stays, need skilled care. Without changing the skilled care requirements, therefore, not all beneficiaries in need will be covered. An approach to fill this gap might be to cover the first 100 or 150 days of a nursing home stay for any Medicare beneficiary. This would encompass those who need skilled care for rehabilitation, but would also offer initial relief to all nursing home residents. Only those with longer stays would have to "spend down" through the Medicaid program. This is effectively the approach suggested by the Pepper Commission (1990). It also could help effectuate a more appropriate transition between acute and long-term care. Under our current system, acute care is sometimes used when that type of care is no longer necessary to compensate for the lack of good long-term care coverage.

On the home health side, benefits could be extended to cover home care services that supplement the medical benefits now offered. This would involve less skilled, homemaker types of services. The requirements for intermittency of the benefit would also need to be relaxed somewhat. This benefit would fill in a gap not now covered consistently under the Medicaid program. But this "moderate" expansion could become a very expensive part of Medicare unless it incorporates time limits and/or cost-sharing requirements. Particularly if nursing home care coverage were limited in duration, the pressures on the

home care side would be great as individuals who ought to be institutionalized tried to remain in the home using these Medicare services.[8] Again, cost sharing might be varied by level of income.

The costs of these two expansions are difficult to predict. When the
costs of the SNF catastrophic benefits were originally estimated, they
were projected to increase spending modestly, costing about $260
million more in 1989—up to about $1.5 billion. In practice, SNF
expanded to $4.5 billion in that year. The net new costs would not be
so great a jump now, since some of the 1989 expansion has been
retained—probably because providers who did not participate before
are now accepting Medicare beneficiaries (Liu and Kenney 1991). But
if the skilled requirement were relaxed, ultimately the level of SNF
use could be substantially higher than that projected for overall SNF
use under the MCCA. Thus, new SNF costs might be much higher—
albeit partially offset by lower Medicaid spending. A full-fledged
home health benefit has been estimated to cost approximately $15
billion for just the elderly in 1990 (Pepper Commission 1990). A more
limited program would cost commensurately less.

How this expansion could be justified and sold politically is a problem, because it runs the risk of being undervalued by beneficiaries in
the same way as the MCCA changes were but would be quite expensive. It might stand a better chance if at least part of the cost was
financed by reducing the comprehensiveness of the acute-care benefit.
Tradeoffs of this kind are discussed in the next section.

Changing the Composition of Medicare Services

Many variations of an approach to reorder Medicare benefits are possible. One option often suggested would be to increase the Part B
deductible and/or premium to pay for expanded long-term care benefits.[9] The long-term care expansion could be all or part of the SNF/
home health changes described previously. SNF and home health
services could be shifted to Part B or to a new Part C, if that is where
the offsetting funding was to be generated. The key issue is how high
the Part B deductible or premium would have to go to fund these
additional benefits.

Since so many beneficiaries now exceed the Part B deductible, raising it just a little will yield considerable savings. As the deductible
amount increases, however, the "return" from this process declines
as fewer and fewer beneficiaries have high enough physician expenses
to go above the deductible. For example, to raise enough revenues to
contribute an average of $500 per year per enrollee for expanded long-

term care would require that the deductible be raised above $1,000. At that level, coverage for acute care places many beneficiaries at considerable risk. To finance a *comprehensive* long-term care plan, the Part B deductible would have to be prohibitively high and combined with Part A increases as well. Thus, this trade-off approach is only viable for small-scale expansions or in combination with a premium increase.

Otherwise, Medicare enrollees would likely turn to the private sector to purchase additional coverage to replace the acute benefit lost. And if the long-term care coverage that this trade-off would support would be less than comprehensive, individuals could end up buying two separate private supplemental policies, each with its own loading and administrative costs. This "solution" would then make financing healthcare even more complicated than it is now. Thus, a trade-off approach alone is an insufficient financing response for anything but small new benefits.

An Optional Long-Term Care Benefit

What about the prospects for saving money by making any added long-term care benefits an optional, and self-financed, part of the program? It makes most sense to think of such a benefit as an insurance program, although some policymakers also have suggested allowing beneficiaries to choose a long-term care track or an acute-care track when they initially enroll in Medicare. Both of these options are briefly considered here.

Offering Public Insurance for Long-Term Care

If no new resources are to be added to Medicare to subsidize long-term care services, why offer a nonsubsidized program? As already mentioned, many individuals are excluded from enrolling in private insurance plans, because they either are too old or have some preexisting medical condition. Thus, one rationale for public insurance is to assure access to individuals through a government insurance program. In addition, Medicare could use its potential market power and its lower administrative costs to make long-term care coverage more affordable to older persons. And it can take a less conservative approach on risks than do private insurers, both because its pool would be very large and because miscalculation of future events could be addressed with later subsidies. Supporters of an optional government program also suggest that it could set the standards for coverage and eligibility against which private insurers would compete. Over time this competition might lead to better products in the private insurance market.

If public insurance were offered in this way to all comers, Medicare might, however, be at a disadvantage as compared to private insurers. What is not clear is whether the increased costs associated with taking all who wish to enroll would be offset by savings from better pooling and lower administrative costs. These two advantages might cancel out the higher costs from adverse selection, but it seems more likely that without some government subsidies, public insurance might still be more expensive than in the private sector if exclusionary practices are allowed that stimulate adverse selection.

The sicker, more disabled population who would be attracted to the public program could be substantial. Each year approximately 180,000 persons who are receiving Social Security disability benefits turn 65. In addition, others who may not have qualified as totally and permanently disabled under Social Security may also have some disability that is likely to result in eligibility for long-term care benefits over time. It would be unfair to prevent such individuals from participating; indeed, giving such persons access to coverage would seem to be a goal of the program. Nonetheless, if these individuals chose the long-term care option, the group could start out with a very adverse risk pool that could quickly escalate costs and discourage others from participating. Private insurers able to exclude such individuals could offer better plans to those in good health, further affecting adverse selection. Thus, even before the program started, it might attract such a poor risk group that it could never be financially viable.

Strict regulations requiring private insurers to take all comers as well would substantially reduce this problem, but might drive most such companies out of business.[10] Thus, if we make optional public insurance viable, it is unlikely that many private insurers would remain in the market. Many consumer advocates are in favor of just such a response, but when optional approaches are discussed, they often pay lip service to retaining the option of buying private insurance.

ALLOWING A TWO-TRACK OPTION UNDER MEDICARE

A second way to make long-term care available on an optional basis would be to allow individuals to choose whether to be on an acute-care "track" or a long-term care "track" under Medicare. The acute-care track would retain the same services now available through Medicare, whereas the long-term track would reduce acute-care benefits in order to extend some long-term care benefits under the program. The major advantage of a two-track approach is that it would allow individuals to choose a different mix of coverage without having to pay more for Medicare.

This type of program could appeal particularly to individuals whose employers or former employers offer supplemental acute-care coverage, but not long-term care insurance. For the working elderly, Medicare is a secondary insurer, so less coverage on the acute-care side and more on the long-term care side would likely mean improved coverage for the worker. Retiree benefits could fill in some of the gaps in acute coverage for those who chose a long-term care option.

A number of critical issues would have to be addressed under such a proposal, including: (1) the trade-offs between acute and long-term care, (2) how frequently, if ever, individuals could switch options after the first election, (3) how the system would be adjusted over time to keep it actuarially fair and financially sound, and (4) whether any beneficiaries would be subsidized to help them afford long-term care coverage.

The first problem is that those who chose a long-term care track would have to forgo considerable acute-care benefits for many years to "buy" the long-term care benefits. For example, the annual premium for even a modest long-term care benefit would total about $600 per year for an average Medicare beneficiary aged 65. As was the case with the trade-off option described earlier, to achieve that solely through changes in the acute-care coverage might require at least a $1,000 Part B deductible and potentially an increase in Part A's deductible as well. Unofficial Congressional Budget Office estimates in 1989 indicated that increasing the Part B deductible to $800 would have freed up only $314 on average to be used for long-term care. And that number is likely to be about the same in 1996 as well. The danger here is that the resulting combination of acute- and long-term care coverage would be inadequate for both types of benefits.

The second problem is that considerable limits would have to be placed on how often, if ever, an individual would be able to switch between the programs, in order to achieve program stability. A one-time-only decision would certainly be the simplest to administer and might result in the least amount of adverse selection. That is, individuals at age 65, most of whom are healthy, would have to decide which plan they wish to participate in so that a reasonable risk pool might result for the long-term care option.[11] More frequent switching—for example, offering the choice every five years—would raise the likelihood of much greater adverse selection, driving up the costs of the program and making it unstable.

The third issue, actuarial fairness, arises because acute health and long-term care insurance represent very different types of insurance risk and require different streams of benefits over time. Payouts under the long-term care option would rise slowly at first, but increase faster in later years. Since the knowledge does not exist to enable the program initially to set an appropriate trade-off between the acute- and long-term care options so as to ensure actuarial fairness, considerable windfalls or shortfalls could be created for Medicare over time, requiring adjustments that could throw the system out of balance. The premium for long-term care insurance might rise much more rapidly than anticipated, for example, generating not only a crisis for Medicare but also for beneficiaries. If prices rise differentially under the two options, this problem could occur even if there were no adverse selection.

Even if the financial balance could be maintained, pressures to expand coverage might be great from individuals in one option who "guessed wrong" to be allowed to switch or at least to receive some relief. In the early years of such a program, pressure would probably come for acute-care relief from those with high deductibles but who are not drawing their long-term care benefits. Later, those in the acute-care option may object when they see their peers receiving long-term care benefits. These pressures might result in allowing switching of options at critical points that could destabilize the financial soundness of Medicare.

Ultimately, the disadvantages of choice outweigh the advantages of moving in this direction. An unstable Medicare program pleasing no one would be the most likely result.

CONCLUSIONS

Stop-loss protection, prescription drug coverage, improved low-income protection, and additional long-term care benefits—each of these areas has been identified in this chapter as worthy of inclusion or expansion under Medicare. But to do any one of these would require a substantial commitment of resources. (To fully evaluate them, we should also consider how they would be financed.)

How do we reconcile simultaneous expansion and contraction? Can cuts in the program exist side by side with increases in other areas? In theory, coordination of these critical goals is possible. The prospects for obtaining so much in savings that both the financial stability of Medicare and limited expansions in the program can be achieved with no added revenues are slim, however. What is more probable is that major cuts will occur along with some reordering of priorities for change. It seems inevitable that beneficiaries will be asked to contribute more for their care, but the composition of that care may not remain the same. A good example of how these two goals could be reconciled is the issue of eligibility age. For example, the eligibility age for Medicare could be reduced, but beneficiaries aged 62 through 67 could be required to pay most of the costs of their own care through higher premiums.

Before making any expansions, it is crucial to establish some priorities. Because of the disparity in the economic status of Medicare beneficiaries, expanding the QMB program should constitute a particularly high priority. Ranking the remaining options for expansion of the acute-care side creates a dilemma: drug coverage is likely to be favored by beneficiaries, whereas many analysts would push for stop-loss protection. This was one of the struggles undertaken in the MCCA where limited expansions in several areas satisfied no one. Drug coverage may be the most difficult for Medicare beneficiaries to obtain elsewhere because of the problems of adverse selection. Since drugs are such an important part of many treatment plans, good care often depends on access to prescription drugs. Moreover, with extended coverage would likely come more oversight of drug pricing, which could be beneficial in other ways as well. Thus, adding prescription drugs to Medicare ought to also rank high.

Regarding long-term care, expanding Medicare to include such care cannot be funded by marginal changes on the acute-care side—the costs are simply too high. Even a limited long-term care program would require a new financing mechanism and should effectively be considered a separate program. For that reason, rather than for the importance of such coverage, it should carry a lower priority.

One of the ironies of the MCCA was that the benefits were criticized as being too insignificant while the costs—at least in terms of higher per enrollee contributions—were faulted for being too high. But the total cost of the benefits offered was essentially equal to the revenues that needed to be raised. The enrollees only wanted the changes if they were cost-free to them. The failed catastrophic legislation proved the difficulty of pleasing both the taxpayers and the beneficiaries who must sign on to any change. What pleases one side may doom a proposal to failure with the other side. Although advocates of change will continue to seek ways to reshape the Medicare program, unless policymakers can become alchemists or unless beneficiaries alter their appreciation for the costs of providing services, this dilemma will not be overcome.

The need to reshape Medicare reaches beyond marginal changes and into the arena of total reform. We can only go so far with incremental expansions; a new healthcare system is needed to facilitate broader changes in Medicare.

Notes

1. This is a less-generous benefit than traditional Medicaid, which covers such non-Medicare services as prescription drugs.

2. This figure assumes that these changes were fully implemented.

3. Medicaid and Medicare are generally not available to these older individuals, unless they have disabilities and qualify for either Supplemental Security Income or Social Security.

4. Spouses and dependents of Medicare beneficiaries under age 65 may also be at risk if they have no independent source of health insurance. If these spouses are not employed or are employed in jobs that offer no insurance, they would only be able to purchase insurance in the individual market.

5. Long-term care could be the subject of a whole book of its own; this discussion merely touches on some of the issues relevant for Medicare. For more discussion of this issue, see Ball (1989); Moon (1989); and Rivlin and Wiener (1988).

6. "Spend down" is a term used to refer to the requirement that before becoming eligible, individuals must spend all of their assets above a certain cutoff to pay for care. Then after becoming asset-eligible, they must spend essentially most of their income each period before Medicaid will pay the balance.

7. The small number of Medicare eligibles compared to patients with other types of financial arrangements seems to be an important factor in nursing homes' decisions to participate in the program, irrespective of payment levels. Moreover, if longer stays were covered and eligibility loosened somewhat, the average cost per day of care for Medicare SNF patients would likely fall, increasing the adequacy of current Medicare payment levels.

8. Criticisms of the current Medicaid program stress the bias toward institutional care that exists, since that part of long-term care services is better funded. The bias in the other direction under Medicare could be even stronger, since most individuals would prefer to remain in their homes if given the choice.

9. Alternatively, a new Part A premium could be introduced. Either way, some adjustments recognizing the need for combining A and B, would be necessary.

10. Another approach would be to develop a less-comprehensive plan—and at considerably lower cost. The public plan could be viewed as a very basic one to give moderate-income individuals better access, rather than competing directly with more generous or comprehensive private insurance offerings. Medicare could carve out one portion of the market, leaving the high end (either as complete packages or supplemental offerings) to the private sector. But again, it would be necessary to set strong standards for the

private market to prevent "cream skimming." Through some type of subsidy, this optional program could also be modestly expanded to those with lower incomes. By putting the coverage in a single package, the pool of persons in a public plan would be increased, probably lessening adverse selection that would occur without any subsidized participation.

11. Another approach might be to only permit a one-time choice but offer some flexibility by allowing individuals to postpone the decision until age 70, for example. In that case, everyone would start out in the traditional Medicare program, but would be able to switch to the long-term care option until they reach age 70. The premium cost and/or deductible trade-off would rise over time to reflect the greater actuarial costs of allowing such a choice.

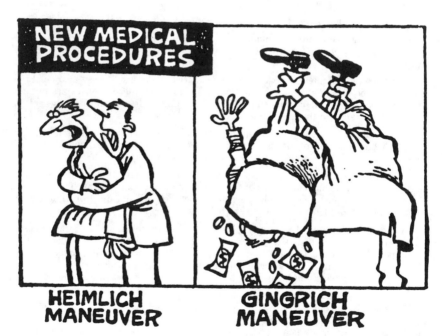

BY MIKE PETERS FOR THE DAYTON DAILY NEWS
USED WITH PERMISSION.

Reprinted with permission of Tribune Media Services.

Chapter Nine

HOW SHOULD MEDICARE CHANGE?

For the debate about the future of Medicare to be most successful, it needs to be guided by what the program was when it began and how it has changed. Medicare's history holds important lessons for its future. Its achievements and its failures constrain future choices and are ignored at society's peril. Bold strokes appeal, but in getting from "here" to where we want to be, we need to understand exactly what "here" is. The bottom line is that it makes sense to maintain Medicare as a separate program for the elderly and disabled, with better coordination of all appropriate parts of healthcare for this group. The only exception would be to fold it into a broader healthcare plan that covers all Americans—which does not seem to be the agenda any time soon.

How should we proceed? We should start out by recognizing a basic tenet of Medicare that is as important today as it was three decades ago. It makes sense both to provide insurance against healthcare expenses and to fund such coverage for elderly and disabled persons largely through contributions by working-age individuals. Americans as individuals have not proven to be farsighted financial planners and are unlikely to save enough during their working years to fund these expenses at retirement. Furthermore, disability often occurs unexpectedly, making insurance protection for this group even more important.

Second, it makes sense to finance the program with contributions that bear a relationship to ability to pay. Although the payroll tax is not progressive, making all wages subject to the tax has resulted in what is effectively a proportional tax.[1] The combination of taxes and benefits is progressive. Moreover, the payroll tax remains a stable and popular source of revenue. Adding any new revenues might more appropriately rely on other sources, but, because of its popularity, the present payroll tax should continue in place.

Third, Americans believe that at least basic healthcare is a right, and Medicare is now a well-established program offering equal access for nearly all elderly and disabled persons so long as they contributed during their working years and "played by the rules." At least for these population groups, universal coverage is thus well accepted. And universal coverage, in turn, offers a number of key advantages.

These elements should be recognized and built upon. But other aspects of Medicare will need to change over time, particularly in the context of fiscal pressures that will surround the program for the foreseeable future. Finally, the failure of broader health system reform efforts creates some specific challenges for Medicare.

FACTORS CONSTRAINING MEDICARE REFORMS

Two challenging constraints place bounds on what can be achieved from Medicare in the foreseeable future. First, financing problems arising from both a history of high rates of healthcare spending growth (not unique to Medicare) and the long-run aging of the population put serious limits on future options for the Medicare program. This, combined with a political climate that precludes much if any reliance on new sources of tax revenue to finance spending, creates pressure for solutions that downsize the program. For the time being, expansions are unlikely unless they are fully funded by elderly and disabled beneficiaries themselves. Promising changes in the program that are fully justifiable in terms of need and program effectiveness— such as covering prescription drugs—are not a serious part of the political agenda at present. And since the demographic pressures on Medicare will begin by the year 2010, there is little time for a change in political will before further financing pressures take root. As a consequence, options that would require more tax revenues are largely eliminated from the ensuing discussion except in the context of a longer term agenda.

Second, the demise of broader healthcare reform makes some desirable changes in Medicare more difficult to make. Expansions in coverage might have been part of such a broader package, although even in the case of the ambitious health reform proposal set forth by the Clinton administration few expansions of Medicare were included. But also at issue is how well Medicare can enforce certain changes if they are limited to just part of the healthcare system. When you push down on one part of the balloon, it simply expands somewhere else. The most obvious example of this is in paying providers. If the rules apply equally across all payers of healthcare, providers cannot shift costs from one source of payment to another.[2] Hospitals, for example, would have to seek greater efficiencies in the provision of care, rather than charging private insurers more to compensate for Medicare's restrictive payments. This would place more stress on providers, but it would also allow more direct control over the impact of payment policies on the efficiency of healthcare delivery.

Similarly, attempts to control the volume of physician services can never be very effective if they only influence a portion of a healthcare professional's business. For example, by limiting allowable increases in the number and intensity of services delivered to Medicare enrollees, the system may do more to encourage physicians to discriminate against the elderly and disabled populations than to change their style of medical practice. Rather than adding discipline to the healthcare market, we would be providing yet another way of gaming the system.

The application of practice guidelines or limits on ineffective treatments would also be substantially more effective if done for the whole population. Since such activities will be most effective if they change the attitudes of both providers and patients, efforts to influence practice must be viewed as systemwide changes and not just as a gimmick by one public program to hold down its own costs. Patients are more likely to accept constraints if they feel they are being equitably applied rather than singling out one group for special treatment. It is easier to make the case that a change will lead to better healthcare if it is applied to everyone. Moreover, it may be easier to change attitudes of younger, healthier individuals than those of the typical Medicare beneficiary, further reducing the potential of reforms aiming to change incentives just among the Medicare population.

The absence of comprehensive health system reform does not mean that Medicare has to proceed completely independently of the rest of the healthcare system. The employer-based insurance market is now aggressively searching for ways to cut costs, putting enormous pressure on healthcare providers to offer increasingly deep discounts. It is even possible that bold moves in this direction by employers, insurance companies, and managed care organizations may effectively shift some costs back onto Medicare. To avoid such an outcome, Medicare must be vigilant in adapting for its own use any cost-saving innovations that may be introduced into the private sector, including any changes in the overall delivery of care that may result from aggressive private sector cost cutting across the board. Even in the absence of comprehensive system reform, coordination between the public and private sectors can at least ensure that the direction of change is consistent throughout the system—essential to avoid continual efforts to shift costs, efforts that do not necessarily save resources for society as a whole.

There is a potential downside to aggressive cost cutting by employers, which may have major consequences for the Medicare program. As part of their cost-cutting efforts, an increasing number of employers are reducing their health insurance offerings. This, combined with failure of universal coverage efforts, suggests that both early retirement coverage before Medicare begins and supplemental coverage after Medicare enrollment may be shrinking. There is already anecdotal evidence of such changes (Foster Higgins 1995). If this trend spreads, it will increase Medicare costs (and increase the beneficiary burden associated with cost sharing and premium increases). It will also increase the numbers left uninsured if the age of eligibility for Medicare is increased—a potentially great source of hardship for many older Americans in the absence of reforms guaranteeing individuals access to private insurance at some price.

Finally, the experience of the 1988 legislative effort to introduce catastrophic coverage makes it clear that asking a relatively small group of high-income elderly and disabled beneficiaries to subsidize the coverage of the poor members of their own age group is politically hazardous. Involving all age groups in any new financing mechanism will make arguments about fairness and the need to share the burden much clearer. In other words, any income-related changes for Medicare are likely to be more successful if they are part of a broader scheme to subsidize protections for low-income groups in the under-65 population as well.

Along similar "fairness" lines, proposals to tax enrollees for part or all of the insurance value of their Medicare benefits make more sense if we also tax the fringe benefits that individuals receive from their employers in the form of health insurance contributions. In the same way that enrollees benefit from the subsidy that Medicare provides, employees receive nonwage compensation from employer-subsidized insurance. It makes little sense to treat one as income but not the other. Both of these proposals are controversial, however, basically for the same reasons. Individuals do not view these in-kind subsidies as income in the same way that tax experts often do. Although taxation of all or part of these benefits may be a viable option for helping finance a comprehensive health system reform, introducing marginal changes in this area simply for deficit-reduction purposes is likely to cause more trouble than it is worth.

These constraints combine to force hard choices for the future of Medicare. The crucial task is to identify which of those choices can improve the program, even in the face of cost constraints, and avoid other choices that would negate the successes of Medicare to date.

One set of productive changes, as outlined here, could be done immediately without waiting for reform elsewhere in the system (many of these were discussed at greater length in chapter 6). On balance, they would result in considerable savings to the federal government and could push back the urgency for more dramatic change. These changes include:

☐ Continue efforts at cost containment involving providers;
☐ Modestly expand the options for managed care;
☐ Revise cost sharing;
☐ Modify the Part B premium to make it income related;
☐ Expand the Qualified Medicare Beneficiary (QMB) program;
☐ Expand the hospice program; and
☐ Streamline billing and administration.

Continue Efforts at Cost Containment Involving Providers

Although Medicare has already relied heavily on reducing payments to providers of services and on payment reforms that alter the incentives for provision of care, more can and should be done in certain provider payment areas. The incentives built into current hospital and physician payment systems now work reasonably well. In the area of hospital payment there is also room for payment reductions, since recent analyses have shown that Medicare is still paying reasonably well as compared to the costs of providing care (ProPAC 1996). Because physician and hospital payments constitute such a large share of Medicare payments, even modest changes in these areas can generate substantial savings over time.

The areas that deserve more attention include home health services, outpatient hospital services, and skilled nursing facility care. Not coincidentally, these are areas where the rate of growth has been disproportionately high over the last few years. Home healthcare in particular is often singled out as a source of overpayment and overuse. These areas will require payment reform in addition to payment reductions. This will take time but should yield substantial savings.

Cost containment efforts must also include better monitoring of service use and better ways of reducing unnecessary care. This is a particular challenge for a fee-for-service system. If, as is likely, the fee-for-service portion of Medicare remains the mechanism that insures the majority of beneficiaries for some time to come, investment in this area is essential. This would require new spending on administrative costs and greater flexibility in regulating service use than is now allowed. A rush to cut costs to Medicare is likely to hurt, rather than help, efforts in this area unless special provisions are made for sufficient funds to improve administrative oversight.

Finally, it is time to separate the cross-subsidies that serve other goals from the Medicare program. At present, Medicare pays for both direct and indirect medical education through its hospital payment system. This artificially inflates the costs of Medicare hospital services and hides the subsidization of medical education from close scrutiny. Another cross subsidy arises in the special disproportionate share payments that Medicare makes to hospitals that treat a high number of indigent patients, not necessarily nor predominantly the elderly or disabled. The entire healthcare system benefits from medical education and relief for indigent care. These costs should not be borne by Medicare alone. At a time when the trust fund that finances Medicare hospital services is facing exhaustion within five years, it is appropriate to finance these activities, worthy though they may be, through programs that make their goals and their subsidization clear. Taking out these subsidies alone would lower the costs of Medicare by about 5 percent.

Modestly Expand Managed Care Options

Although managed care under Medicare has lagged considerably below the growth in the private sector, it now serves 10 percent of all beneficiaries. In the interests of offering the same options to beneficiaries as are available to other age groups, it is important to continue to foster managed care development within the Medicare program. Recent moves by the Health Care Financing Administration to relax plan restrictions will likely help to expand HMO participation under Medicare. But, there are several reasons for taking a go-slow approach. First, Medicare would do well to learn from the experiences (mistakes and successes) now taking place in managed care for the under-65 population. Second, Medicare HMO experience to date suggests that ill-considered expansion in this area may not save any money for the federal government. In particular, the way in which the Medicare program pays premiums on behalf of beneficiaries needs to be over-hauled. Medicare pays a premium equal to the cost of an average beneficiary, a formula that has several disadvantages. It ties payments to fee-for-service when the claim of managed care is that it can and should do better than fee-for-service. In addition, even though the HMO payment amount is set at 95 percent of the fee-for-service rate, the rate of growth in the payment matters more than the level. Further, because Medicare uses only a crude adjustment for differences in the health status of beneficiaries, it loses money on the HMO option if, as is likely, this option attracts healthier than average beneficiaries (or just those who choose to use fewer services). Medicare pays more than the costs of serving the HMO enrollees, yet is left with disproportion-ate numbers of expensive beneficiaries in the fee-for-service part. Only a small amount of such adverse risk selection is enough to put the program seriously out of balance. Reform of the payment structure should precede steps to encourage many more beneficiaries to enroll in the HMO option.

A first step in payment reform would flow naturally from the pro-posal to eliminate medical education and disproportionate share pay-ments from hospital services (described above). Since those payments are now implicitly in the premiums paid to HMOs, and since HMOs effectively do not share these subsidies with the hospitals performing medical education or helping indigent patients, such subsidies rep-resent an overpayment to HMOs that would be instantly eliminated. If not taken out of the fee-for-service side, however, an explicit reduc-tion in the HMO premium should be made.

Second, Medicare needs to find ways to tie the growth of payments to HMOs to something other than the fee-for-service part of Medicare. Growth in the costs of managed care elsewhere might be one option; another would be overall healthcare costs. Experimentation with com-petitive bidding for Medicare HMO contracts could also be tried. The important factor is to allow sufficient growth to foster reasonable cov-erage and treatment while seeking federal savings.

A third reason for a go-slow approach in the HMO context is the need for careful assessment of risk adjustors. Until an effective risk adjustment system can be developed, it is crucial to limit the range of private options, which tend to be dividers of the risk pool. That is, if options were offered that appeal more to healthier individuals (such as medical savings accounts), the chances of overpayment to such plans would be very high and the costs to Medicare would be very large. Greater flexibility and choice should only occur after this basic issue for Medicare is successfully resolved. Otherwise, the advantage of a large universal risk pool for Medicare will be lost and the federal government will pay dearly for that loss.

Finally, Medicare also needs to develop effective ways to monitor the quality of care of HMO plans to ensure that beneficiaries are adequately protected. This is essential, particularly because Medicare beneficiaries will not have the same types of oversight protections that employer-subsidized plans often have through benefits managers and other advocates who can intervene on behalf of enrollees when problems arise. Work in this area is still underdeveloped.

Revise Cost Sharing

We ought to bring a better balance and logic to Medicare's cost sharing. This could be done while achieving modest savings, but it is important to consider these changes in concert with increases in the premium and expansions in low income projections. The most important reductions in cost sharing should be the elimination of hospital coinsurance, limiting the Part A deductible, and reductions in skilled nursing facility (SNF) coinsurance. Expansions to offset these changes would come in an increase in the Part B deductible and potentially adding a modest home health coinsurance. Further, shifting home healthcare from Part A to Part B would make it subject to the Part B premium and deductible, further increasing cost sharing.

Hospital coinsurance and multiple deductibles do little to discourage unnecessary use of services, particularly given the other strong controls on hospital use in the Medicare program. Rather, these cost-sharing mechanisms are essentially used to cut federal costs by shifting the burdens onto beneficiaries. The hospital deductible is considerably higher than that normally found in the private sector. And the coinsurance is not only inordinately high, but it unnecessarily complicates the program. It does not begin until after 60 days; individuals with such long hospital stays (or multiple stays) are unlikely to be in a position to respond to economic incentives. Further, hospital cost sharing is based on an arbitrary spell-of-illness concept, which was adopted as a means for limiting costs in the program and not based on any sound medical rationale.

SNF coinsurance largely limits the program to a 20-day benefit rather than a 100-day benefit because of high coinsurance rates. Since the coinsurance is linked to the costs of hospital care, it bears no relationship to costs of providing skilled nursing care. Adopting a 20 percent coinsurance for SNF would improve the consistency of the benefit and, if applied to all days, would not raise Medicare costs (CBO 1995a).

Reductions in Part A cost sharing could be offset with an increase in the Part B deductible, since, at $100 per year, this part of Medicare's cost sharing is low relative to the private sector. Raising the Part B deductible and indexing it over time might also discourage unnecessary use of routine physician visits. Thus, this deductible might not only require beneficiaries to pay more, but it might be a tool to influence use of services—actually achieving the stated goal of cost sharing.

Another change that would result in substantial savings to the Medicare program would be to shift the home health services benefit fully into Part B from Part A. Originally, Medicare home healthcare was split between the two parts of the program. As an ambulatory service, it is arguably more appropriate for Part B, leaving Part A solely as institutional care. But a more important argument for the purposes here is that home health would then be subject both to the deductible and to calculation of the Part B premium. Together these would constitute a substantial increase in the share beneficiaries are asked to contribute to the Medicare program. Over one-fourth of the costs of this benefit would then be paid by beneficiaries.

A second change affecting beneficiaries would require a modest copayment for each visit. As described earlier in this chapter and in chapter 3, home health services have averaged growth rates well in excess of 20 percent in the 1990s. At least part of this growth almost certainly represents abuses by providers to offer more services than beneficiaries would choose if they were required to share in the costs. In fact, many beneficiaries may be unaware of the extent of the services they receive or their costs. If the copayment were moderate—say $5 per visit—it would not be very much of a burden, but would make patients much more aware of the services they were receiving. In making the change, care is necessary to avoid undue burdens on the small group with substantial needs for care. For this reason, combining the shift to Part B and the modest copayment would be a fairer approach than imposing a large coinsurance (say, 20 percent). As with all these changes, a critical additional piece is protection for beneficiaries with low and moderate incomes.

A number of combinations of changes in Part A and B are reasonable, but I would restrict cost sharing in the hospital to no more than one deductible per year (or institute a premium in lieu of the deductible), initially set that deductible at about $500, eliminate hospital coinsurance, and reduce the SNF coinsurance to 20 percent of the costs of SNF care (about $20 per day in 1992). The Part B deductible could be increased to $350 per year to offset most of the costs of the Part A changes. The net costs of this change would be less than $0.5 billion—an amount that could be made up with the premium changes described in the next section.

One complication of raising the federal government's liabilities under Part A and reducing them under Part B would be a worsening of the Part A trust fund balances. For this and other reasons, it is appropriate to combine these two parts of the program and make explicit decisions about how much of the additional revenues for Medicare (over and above the payroll contributions) should come from premiums and how much from general revenues. Short of that, shifting home health services to Part B would ease the situation.

Expand the Part B Premium

Another element in rebalancing beneficiary contributions under Medicare would be to expand the Part B premium and add an income-related piece. Beneficiaries should be asked to contribute more for their care, but in a way that protects those with few resources. It also should deemphasize any welfare stigma in doing so. These two goals raise considerable practical problems, however.[3]

A wide range of options are possible (as described earlier) to raise the Part B premium. Without adding a new administrative structure, however, the most feasible approaches are to either adopt across-the-board increases in premiums or generate an income-related premium using the income tax structure. Although this was extremely unpopular when combined with the expansions of benefits in the catastrophic legislation of the late 1980s, politicians from both political parties have since embraced, at least in theory, the concept of an income-related premium—and although efforts have often been made to avoid using the income tax—it remains the most practical.

Part A of Medicare implicitly has had an income-related premium since 1994. At that time, taxation of Social Security benefits was extended so that high-income individuals and couples now are required to include 85 percent of their Social Security benefits in income for purposes of calculating income taxes. This is up from counting 50 percent as taxable income for persons with incomes above $32,000 and $44,000 for singles and couples, respectively. The revenues from raising the amount subject to taxation from 50 to 85 percent are now dedicated to the Part A trust fund, making it an income-related payment from Social Security beneficiaries toward the cost of their own medical care. In 1996, this adds about $4 billion going to the Part A trust fund (HI Trustees 1996). This concept could be expanded, or a separate income-related premium established for Part B. Expansion could involve adding a portion of the benefits received by older and disabled persons from Medicare as part of individual incomes. While this is likely the most equitable approach (CBO 1994), it would involve a major change that has potential implications for taxation of employee fringe benefits. A less intrusive approach would be to combine an across-the-board increase in the Part B premium with a new income-related supplement to it.

As described in chapter 7, there simply are not enough high-income older and disabled persons to raise a large amount of revenue without also increasing the basic premium unless the cutoff is set relatively low—i.e. below $50,000 for couples. Only about 6 percent of older persons reside in families with incomes above $75,000 (U.S. Bureau of the Census 1995d). And the share of disabled persons with such incomes is likely to be even lower. But if the cutoff is very low, the concept of asking "high-income" beneficiaries to pay more is quickly lost. As a matter of equity, however, it may be good policy to raise the Part B premium on even a small number of high-income individuals to a level well above the basic premium. The appropriate balance could be fine-tuned over time.

If home health services are also shifted from Part A of the program to Part B, that change will increase premium liabilities substantially as well. This makes it important to raise the basic level slowly. An initial increase to 27 percent in combination with the Part A shift would increase the premium in 1996 from its current level of $42.50 to $57.40 per month, for example.

Expand the QMB Program

Improved protection for those with low and moderate incomes should occur simultaneously with changes in cost sharing. The QMB program now pays the premiums, deductibles, and coinsurance of Medicare beneficiaries whose incomes are below poverty. It also covers premiums for those between 100 and 120 percent of poverty under the related Specified Low Income Medicare Beneficiary Program (SLMB).[4] QMB protection should extend higher up the income scale than just to 120 percent of the poverty line. That is, it should reduce the cost-sharing burdens for more than just the poor. Those with modest incomes now have difficulty paying this cost sharing, which reduces their access to the program. Initially, persons with incomes below at least 150 percent of poverty should be protected at least for premium payments—with further expansions potentially added later.

This additional protection for cost sharing under Medicare ought to be part of the Medicare program, shifting the QMB program out of Medicaid. This would help ensure that beneficiaries would participate in the QMB program and that QMB would be a full-fledged part of Medicare. Many beneficiaries either are unaware of the program or are reluctant to apply for it through Medicaid. This shift would also help ease some of the pressures on Medicaid, but to keep the costs low initially, it might need to be done in stages.

These changes would raise the costs to the federal government by about $5 billion to $6 billion. Some of this would come from shifting to the federal government burdens now placed on the states through Medicaid, some from increased participation from eligibles likely if QMB is part of Medicare, and part from expanding protection to those up to 150 percent of poverty.

The combined impact of these three changes—modest expansion of cost sharing, expansion of the Part B premium, and expansion of the QMB program—would result in net savings for the Medicare program of nearly $7 billion to $8 billion in 1996, combined with a more equitable cost-sharing framework. It would recognize the income and health diversity of Medicare beneficiaries—that is, the need to protect some beneficiaries while asking higher contributions of others—and do so in a way that is perceived as fairer and less drastic than the catastrophic changes proposed in 1988.

Expand the Hospice Program

Changes in the hospice program to raise its status as an acceptable mainstream alternative to more aggressive types of treatment at the end of life could be done at little additional cost to Medicare by easing current restrictions on hospice coverage. Providers could be encouraged to participate rather than be subjected to the stringent requirements now on the books. Some of the changes would be largely symbolic; others would attract more patients and save costs elsewhere in the Medicare system. Some resources could be spent to promote hospice care—for example, by funding demonstrations to stress that this is a reasonable choice and one that is easy for patients to make.

This effort ought to be combined with an aggressive effort to educate patients and their families about alternatives and choices. Promotion of living wills and of durable powers of attorney that allow Medicare enrollees to make their wishes known could be coordinated with these efforts. Too often, less care is associated with inferior care or a withdrawal of support. Attitudes of patients, families, and providers about alternatives need to change. These education efforts should focus on *choice* and not on requirements for types of care. In addition, Medicare should experiment further with ways to promote flexibility in benefits covered at the end of life. For example, full coverage of prescription drugs used by outpatients might be one way to expand protections for those who wish to remain at home at the end of their lives.

Streamline Billing and Administration

A low-cost change that could substantially improve Medicare in the eyes of both beneficiaries and providers would be to simplify billing and administration of the program. The cost-sharing changes outlined above would help ease some of the complexity of the program, but streamlining should go further.

While doctors are now required to file for patients, patients can still be asked to pay upfront for services, so that billing remains complicated. Further, patients may lose track of the services they have received. Coordination of bills with private insurers could also help. Finally, the complexity of the "Explanation of Medicare Benefits" forms that beneficiaries receive has long been a source of legitimate complaint.

One solution would be for beneficiaries to receive one bill quarterly or bimonthly, allowing them to pay just once for any cost sharing owed. Clear language would indicate what Medicare contributes— helping to underscore the substantial amount that Medicare provides—and what is paid by private insurers. This would have the additional benefit of reminding enrollees how much of the total bill Medicare (as opposed to Medigap) actually pays, and helping them identify problem or fraudulent billing. Streamlining the billing process could eventually lead to substantial administrative savings, in terms of both lower spending when less paperwork is needed, and saved time and frustration for both patients and healthcare providers. If Medicare can truly claim that it reduces those burdens, future payment cuts will certainly be more palatable as well. It is likely that any costs incurred in making these changes could be recouped with lower payments elsewhere in the system. Further, Medicare needs to streamline its data reporting for its own internal purposes, with benefits to beneficiaries and providers a fortunate by-product.

LONGER TERM STEPS

The challenges in finding savings to keep the current Medicare program healthy into the future will occupy the attention of policymakers for years to come. Even if healthcare spending can be brought into line with the rate of growth of GDP, the aging of the population will likely necessitate both the increases in beneficiary contributions outlined above and further contributions after 2010. Further restructuring of the program or adoption of private sector innovations may be appropriate over time as well. But, at some point it will also be essential to consider an increase in the contribution from payroll or other broad-based taxes to finance healthcare for an increasing share of the population. Aside from reforms that increase the efficiency of the delivery of services, all of the options to keep Medicare sound implicitly represent financing issues: the question is who will pay and when.

Further, this section on long-run solutions to the problems facing Medicare focuses on some increases in direct financing and some options for modest expansions in the program that could be financed largely by the beneficiaries themselves. While these are not popular pieces of the puzzle at present, they ought to be given serious consideration at some point in the future.

Further Reform Medicare to Address Costs of Healthcare

Until some of the short-run changes in Medicare to slow the growth in spending have been made, and some of the uncertainty surrounding changes currently going on in health service delivery and the private insurance market is resolved, exactly what next steps are appropriate for Medicare will remain a question. If some of the reforms described above begin to slow Medicare growth to more reasonable levels, as is plausible, less restructuring or other changes might be needed over time. And if private initiatives prove able to slow the rate of growth of healthcare spending substantially, Medicare can take advantage of that experience with further moves into private options. Despite claims by some that we have found the needed solutions to healthcare spending growth, experimentation and further modifications of new approaches are likely for some time to come.

It is also important to distinguish which types of changes will actually slow the growth in healthcare spending and which will merely shift the cost burden to individuals and families. For example, vouchers can save the federal government money by limiting its liabilities under Medicare to a fixed per capita amount. But if vouchers do not lead to greater efficiency (by encouraging greater cost sensitivity by beneficiaries), then the problem will not be resolved, it will simply be passed on to individuals. It would simply "individualize" the problem rather than treat it as a shared concern. Moving it out of the public sector does not eliminate the problem; instead it becomes only an indirect way to increase costs to beneficiaries. This point needs to be made clearly and forcefully in the public debate.

Increasing Direct Costs to Beneficiaries

Passing further costs of the program on to beneficiaries beyond what might occur in the near term needs to be carefully balanced against beneficiary ability to absorb these costs (and assessed in the context of other benefit changes such as those in Social Security). This balance can be analyzed in a relatively straightforward way for proposals such as increased premiums or cost sharing. Per capita impacts can be estimated and then compared to the income levels of the individuals who would be affected. Shifting the burden to individuals through vouchers or raising the age of Medicare eligibility will be more subtle in its impact and less easy to assess in terms that are clearly communicable in the public debate.

Vouchers in the form of fixed dollar payments to beneficiaries give flexibility to those whose own incomes are high enough for the vouchers to be an effective facilitator of choice among insurance options. But if the voucher's insurance buying power shrinks over time, more and more beneficiaries will find the voucher too little to make any real difference to their choices. Because of the regressive nature of a flat amount voucher and the elimination of public concern for the costs of care that a voucher engenders, this is not the best long-run strategy.

Raising the age of eligibility for Medicare, on the other hand, deserves a serious look in the context of the difficult choices the aging of the population will necessitate. But, it comes with a number of disadvantages. First, without reform of the private insurance market, those out of the labor force may find it difficult to obtain insurance—and raising the eligibility age will increase the size of this vulnerable group. At a minimum, allowing older workers to buy into the Medicare program at reasonable actuarial levels would be important.[5] A higher eligibility age will also burden employers who now offer retiree benefits (and their retirees), because they would have to fill in the insurance gaps for a longer period before Medicare eligibility would begin. Employers will face strong incentives to cut back on such benefits in the face of higher burdens. If, as a consequence of raising the eligibility age, the number of uninsured rises (placing burdens on public hospitals), the costs of producing goods and services rise (to cover greater retiree health benefits), and the number of young families who must help support their older relatives increases, we will be just as burdened as a society as we were before. We will not have solved anything. The costs will simply not show up on the ledgers of the federal government.

Increase Public Financing for Medicare

Ultimately, additional public funds will almost certainly be required to cover Medicare's long-run costs. Although the taxable base for Medicare has increased in recent years and some revenues from the taxation of Social Security benefits are bolstering the trust fund, Medicare will both implicitly (in the general revenue financing for Part B) and explicitly (from the payroll tax base of Part A) require further federal revenues. And this is appropriate. As the numbers of beneficiaries grow from about 14.3 percent of the population in 1996 to about 18.4 percent of the population in 2020 and even higher in later years, both the share of GDP and of the federal budget devoted to Medicare should rise simply to keep pace with demographic change. At the same time, the share of the population getting insurance from other sources will fall, at least partially offsetting higher costs to Medicare—a fact often ignored by those who talk about the "unacceptable" level of Medicare as compared to the rest of the federal budget.

It should also be kept in mind that the payroll tax share of Medicare, at 2.9 percent (reflecting the combined employer and employee amounts) of earnings, has not risen since 1986 (HI Trustees 1996). It remains only a small part of the FICA total of 15.3 percent of payroll. If the percentage of payroll devoted to Medicare were increased by a factor just large enough to account for the growth in the share of the population who benefit from the program, the tax rate would need to be about 3.2 percent by 2000 and over 4 percent by 2020. And some further allowance might be needed to cover growth in the costs of healthcare. Similar factors might be applied to general revenues to meet needs for Part B but to also keep the spending growth from expanding too rapidly.

Thus, even if Medicare were to achieve substantial savings in the provision of basic benefits, and even if beneficiaries were required to pay more, moderate increases in payroll or other taxes will have to be considered. The types of changes suggested above do not imply allowing tax growth to "get out of hand"; rather these changes should seem quite reasonable to the average taxpayer.

Improve Acute-Care Coverage

Expansion of Medicare to cover prescription drugs or preventive services, or to provide stop-loss protection, could best be done in the context of standards of coverage for the population as a whole.[6] In other words, we need some consensus on a national minimum insurance coverage, even though many younger Americans have more generous coverage than what such a minimum would be, and even though the cost of such coverage would be higher for the elderly and disabled than for other groups.

Prescription drugs are one of the important benefits that need to be viewed in this context. Drugs are an important part of the treatment of many health problems, and lack of coverage can lead to poor health outcomes and ultimately higher costs. But for the elderly in particular, the costs of prescription drugs are high and would increase the costs of Medicare substantially. Further, although stop-loss protection was undervalued by the elderly when it was covered by the MCCA, it is part of any insurance program that seeks to limit risks of catastrophic expenditures and should be provided under Medicare. For Medicare beneficiaries, an individual limit of $4,000 or $5,000 could suffice, *if* low-income persons are protected from the cost-sharing burden.

These two benefit expansions—prescription drugs and stop loss— could be offered as an optional Part C of Medicare, fully funded by the premiums charged. (A subsidized version could also be developed for those with moderate or low incomes.) When combined with the improvements in cost sharing described above, this could constitute a basic Medigap package, largely replacing the expensive and relatively inefficient Medigap coverage that is now sold privately. Without specific controls on who could buy such insurance, however, Medicare might suffer from the kinds of adverse selection discussed throughout the book, particularly since this package would be associated with the fee-for-service option under Medicare. One option might be to require that this be the only Medigap package that a beneficiary could purchase under Medicare. Those who wish more generous packages would buy them privately. With appropriate structuring of the privately marketed packages, this might reduce the risk selection that could otherwise occur.

Expand Long-Term Care Coverage

Improved long-term care coverage for the elderly and disabled makes sense on several grounds. First, the current system of relying on Medicaid and individuals' own resources results in great hardships and inequities. Long-term care coverage could substantially improve the quality of life of many who now do without needed care or get by with less than optimal care. Second, the problem of long-term care is amenable to a shared-risk approach, which is missing from our current system. Third, the acute-care system is currently misused to compensate for the much better coverage available for acute-care problems than for long-term care. Medicare is the major insurer affected by this misuse and has higher costs because of it.

But even an income-related long-term care program will be expensive. It is not feasible to fully fund it by shifting resources from Medicare or even from Social Security—although this could certainly be part of the financing scheme. It must be funded at least in part with public revenues. The elderly and disabled populations can and should be asked to pay a substantial share of any new burdens from expanding long-term care. But since these burdens are now shared with the young, the young should also help to support such programs.

Several approaches are possible. I favor a comprehensive program of nursing home and community-based care with substantial, but income-related, cost sharing. Those who can afford to do so would be asked to pay much, but not all, of the costs of their care. This would give them a stake in the program and ensure that all or most care falls under a system that can be subjected to cost controls. Other approaches, such as that offered by the Pepper Commission (1990) or mandatory insurance coverage where people pay premiums on a sliding scale, could also achieve the goals of protection for disabled people, and at a lower price than that of full social insurance.

But any of these limited approaches will still result in a substantial increase in tax burdens for Americans—perhaps in the range of $50 billion to $60 billion annually.[7] At this point such a target remains only a wish. It is unlikely to become reality in the foreseeable future, particularly as long as many younger families remain uninsured for acute-care needs.

CONCLUSIONS

Expectations for improving the Medicare program from the perspective of its beneficiaries have declined since the first part of the 1990s. The failure to pass expanded health coverage for Americans and the current antitax, antigovernment sentiment militates against expansion. Indeed, much of our focus for the near future will likely be on restraining growth in the program.

Changes can be made in the system, however. Improved cost-sharing requirements, some increase in premiums, better low-income protections, improved administration, and an expanded hospice program are all consistent with a less expansive system. Indeed, it is crucial to seek these reforms rather than settle for cuts that only have budgetary goals.

The more difficult challenge is to envision broader changes that could further improve the program. The problems of affordability of health services, the need to better coordinate care, and the importance of sharing the financing of care for retired and disabled persons will not go away simply because the population is aging. Over the next decade Medicare will face extraordinary pressures for change. It is not necessary that all of these represent a shrinking of protection.

Notes

1. In 1993, legislation eliminated the cap on what is subject to taxation for Medicare.

2. Obviously the simplest form of coordination would be through a single program with a single administrative entity overseeing the system. But so-called all-payer systems could also provide coordination in a world of multiple insurers. What would be required is regulation that requires all of these payers to play by the same rules.

3. The simplest way to introduce a sliding scale premium would be to use the Social Security system. Part B premiums are already taken out of individuals' checks, and that could be continued. But instead of a flat payment, the premium could be tied to the size of the Social Security benefit. This could work on a sliding scale up to a cap. After exploring this approach, however, it becomes clear that there is not enough variation in Social Security benefits to achieve a truly progressive premium. This is likely to be useful only as a means for providing some protection for those with low benefit amounts.

4. For purposes of this discussion QMB and SLMB are combined since they are so closely related as protections for those with low incomes.

5. But this could also create costs for Medicare if those who could get less expensive insurance because they are good risks buy it in the private sector, leaving Medicare with only high-cost individuals.

6. This is not to say that coverage has to be identical. For example, if appropriate medical care requires more visits for well babies and less screening for other groups of the population, then differences could be established. But the standards ought to be based on appropriateness or effectiveness and not on source of insurer.

7. Such estimates are subject to enormous variation and, not surprisingly, are very controversial. The Pepper Commission (1990) proposal carried an estimated price tag of $42.8 billion in 1990 dollars. That amount would be considerably higher if expressed in 1996 dollars.

APPENDIX

THE MECHANICS OF MEDICARE

The Medicare program was established by legislation in 1965 as Title XVIII of the Social Security Act and first went into effect on July 1, 1966.[1] The program is divided into two basic parts: Part A is Hospital Insurance (also referred to as HI), and Part B is Supplementary Medical Insurance (SMI).

Eligibility

Medicare covers three groups of individuals: persons aged 65 or over who are also eligible for any type of Social Security benefit, persons who have been receiving Social Security disability benefits for two years, and insured workers, their spouses, or children with end-stage renal disease (ESRD). Dependents and widows or widowers of retired workers are covered, so long as they are at least age 65. Disability coverage is limited to the covered worker or an adult disabled child of a covered worker. Eligible persons are enrolled in Medicare Part A at no charge.

When Medicare was first passed in 1965, it covered only elderly persons, and initially everyone over the age of 65 was eligible. That blanket eligibility included all persons who reached age 65 by 1968. Consequently, all persons aged 93 and over in 1996 have Medicare coverage regardless of their Social Security status. Subsequently, only those over age 65 who were eligible for some type of Social Security benefit were eligible for Medicare. But even without blanket coverage, over 98 percent of all persons aged 65 and over are covered by Medicare either as a worker or dependent. In 1996, approximately 33.4 million elderly persons were enrolled in the Medicare program.

Anyone over the age of 65 who is not otherwise eligible may elect to enroll in Medicare by paying an actuarially fair premium. That premium was $289 per month in 1996, and about 304,000 persons elected such enrollment. These are generally persons who have had little or no labor force attachment or who have immigrated to the United States from other countries and lived here for at least five years. For persons with substantial workforce experience but who do not have enough credits to fully qualify, legislation in 1993 created a new lower premium for those with 30 to 39 quarters of coverage. In 1996, this premium is $188 per month.

The two-year waiting period for Medicare coverage for disabled persons, coupled with a five-month waiting period for eligibility for Social Security, means that individuals with disabilities do not receive Medicare coverage until 29 months after the onset of the disability. They may also continue to receive benefits for up to 36 months after Social Security cash benefits end, so long as they are still disabled. Persons disabled as children may also qualify once they reach age 18 if their parents were eligible for Social Security. In 1996, 4.6 million disabled persons were covered by Medicare. Dependents of disabled beneficiaries are not eligible for Medicare unless they are age 65 or older.

ESRD patients are covered once they file for benefits and if they are entitled to monthly Social Security benefits or are children or spouses of covered workers. In 1996, there were approximately 244,000 ESRD beneficiaries.

All persons enrolled in Part A of Medicare and all persons over the age of 65 may also elect to join Part B, which requires a monthly premium contribution to pay some of the costs of the Part B benefits. When persons enroll in Medicare or turn age 65, the Part B premium is automatically deducted from their monthly Social Security check. Enrollees must inform the Social Security Administration if they do not want to enroll in Part B. If an eligible individual elects to delay joining Part B, a penalty (of 10 percent for each year of delay) is added to the premium to discourage individuals from joining only when they are sicker. (The premium is discussed later in this appendix.)

The generosity of the subsidy means that most, but not all, join. Most elderly beneficiaries elect this option, but a smaller percentage of disabled persons do so. In 1994, over 96 percent of elderly and 90 percent of disabled Part A beneficiaries elected Part B coverage.

Legislation in the 1980s made Medicare the secondary payer in cases where enrollees aged 65 to 69 were still in the labor force and had private health insurance. The private insurance company is liable for the bulk of acute-care expenses, and Medicare will pay only for services not covered by this private insurance. Although this provision has been poorly enforced, in theory it limits eligibility for working enrollees. An individual may decline to take private coverage from an employer, for example, if a large premium contribution is required. In that case, the worker would receive full benefits from Medicare.

Yet another dimension of eligibility is the creation of Qualified Medicare Beneficiaries (QMBs) under the Medicare Catastrophic Coverage Act (MCCA) of 1988. These special beneficiaries, whose incomes must be below 100 percent of the federal poverty level and whose resources are under twice the amount specified for Supplemental Security Income, are entitled to have the Medicaid program pick up the costs of Medicare's premium, deductibles, and coinsurance. Although most of the MCCA was repealed in 1989, this provision remained in force. These protections were partially expanded under the Omnibus Budget Reconciliation Act (OBRA) of 1990. Beneficiaries can have Medicaid pay for their Part B premiums if their incomes are between 100 percent and 120 percent of poverty under the related Specified Low Income Medicare Beneficiary (SLMB) program. Thus far, only a portion of those eligible for QMB or SLMB protection have signed up; many beneficiaries seem to be unaware of the programs.

Benefits

Medicare coverage is limited to acute-care services, particularly physician services and acute hospital care. This basic benefit package has changed little since Medicare's inception.

PART A

Under Part A, hospital coverage is limited to 90 days within a "spell of illness," plus a one-time supply of 60 "lifetime reserve days" that can be used to extend the covered period within one or more spells of illness. The first 60 days of the spell of illness are fully covered (after payment of a deductible). After that, the beneficiary is liable for coinsurance for the next 30 days (see the discussion upcoming).[3] The lifetime reserve days, which would then begin, also require beneficiary cost sharing. A spell of illness begins when the patient receives hospital or extended care services and ends when 60 days have elapsed between such periods of treatment. Thus, a spell of illness is not really related to a particular illness, but, rather, refers to a period of time elapsing before the next spell begins. Inpatient psychiatric services are limited to 190 days over a patient's lifetime.

Another Part A benefit is skilled nursing facility (SNF) care for up to 100 days in a qualified facility per spell of illness. This is a very limited benefit, however, that must follow a three-day period of hospitalization and is restricted to enrollees who require the skills of

technical or professional personnel for skilled nursing or rehabilitation. This is not a general nursing home benefit, but is intended to be
an extension of acute-care treatment. Coinsurance is charged beginning on the 21st day of the stay.[4]

Home health, like SNF, is a restricted benefit, largely provided under
Part A.[5] Coverage is limited to skilled nursing or rehabilitation benefits provided in the home. Unlike SNF, no prior hospitalization is
required, and there is no limit on the number of days that can be
covered. But home health services must be prescribed by a physician
with the expectation of rehabilitation for the patient. The care must
be "intermittent," usually defined as less than daily, but recent guidelines permit a period of daily visits of up to eight hours per day.
Finally, the patient must be confined to the home—a requirement
somewhat at odds with the stipulation that the care received be
intermittent.[6]

Hospice care was added to Part A as a benefit in 1983. It includes
nursing care, physical and occupational therapy, medical social services, home health aide services, continuous home care if necessary,
medical supplies, physicians' services, short-term inpatient care, and
counseling. Persons electing hospice benefits face limitations on what
other Medicare services are covered that relate to the terminal illness,
however. For example, if a person elects to be in the hospice program,
only inpatient care for alleviation of pain, respite care, or acute symp-
tom management is permitted. Aggressive treatment for the terminal
illness would not be covered. A physician must certify that the patient
is terminally ill and is expected to die within six months. After an
initial eligiblity period of 210 days, benefits may be extended for a
final period of unlimited duration if patients are recertified by their
doctors. Services must be performed by a certified hospice program
and must reflect a written plan of care.

PART B

Part B of Medicare pays 80 percent of physicians' "reasonable"
charges (also called "allowed" charges) for surgery, consultation, and
home, office, and institutional visits after the enrollee meets a $100
deductible. These reasonable charges are established by a complex
payment calculation that was replaced in 1992 by the Medicare Fee
Schedule (discussed in chapter 3). Routine physicals are not covered.
Restrictions are placed on certain nonphysician providers of care such
as dentists, chiropractors, and podiatrists. Mental health services are
also limited to 62.5 percent of actual service costs. In addition, copayments and deductibles are charged. Other covered services include

x-ray and radiation therapy, ambulance services, physical and speech therapy, and rural health clinic services. Physicians are also permitted, although within strict limits, to charge beneficiaries more than the reasonable amounts established by Medicare—a practice referred to as "balance billing" (described in more detail later here).

Part B also covers 80 percent of the reasonable charges for diagnostic tests, home dialysis supplies, durable medical equipment, and artificial devices. The budget summit of 1990 also added biennial mammography screening coverage, and influenza shots have been covered since 1993.

Facility charges for hospital outpatient services and ambulatory surgery centers are also covered, again with coinsurance requirements.[7] An individual treated in a hospital outpatient department or emergency room or an ambulatory surgery center will receive at least two bills—one for the facility and one for the physician.

HMOs

Medicare also allows its beneficiaries to enroll in health maintenance organizations (HMOs) and similar organizations called "competitive medical plans" that meet certain conditions. The HMO must provide all the services that Medicare covers. The Medicare program pays the HMO directly for the costs of the beneficiary according to a formula designed to pay 95 percent of the benefit payments for a similar beneficiary in the fee-for-service portion of Medicare, referred to as the adjusted average per capita cost (AAPCC). Beneficiaries who wish to participate must enroll in Part B. The HMO may charge a premium in lieu of the deductibles and coinsurance amounts the beneficiary would pay if not in the HMO. The HMO premium may also be higher to cover services beyond what Medicare normally provides. For example, some HMOs offer prescription drug coverage. Beneficiaries electing to enroll in a Medicare-approved HMO must abide by the rules of the HMO and will not be covered for any services performed outside the rules established by the HMO, but they may disenroll at any time. Beneficiaries do not have to file any claims forms. HMOs are at risk if the costs of care exceed their AAPCC payments, and they must share at least part of any savings with beneficiaries in the form of improved benefits. In 1996, some restrictions on plans were eased, allowing plans to offer beneficiaries the option of going outside the plan for some services.

Once a very limited part of Medicare, the HMO program has been expanding rapidly in recent years. In late 1995, 3.8 million beneficiaries were enrolled.

Cost Sharing and Premiums

Enrollees in the Medicare program are required to share some of the costs of their own care—both through a premium for coverage under Part B and payment of a portion of the costs of services received in the form of deductibles and coinsurance. Most of these contributions grow each year as healthcare costs increase under Medicare. All enrollees (not in HMOs) are liable for these payments, although Medicaid pays for certain low-income enrollees, and others may receive or purchase private insurance to cover these liabilities.

PART A

For Part A, this cost sharing is organized around the concept of "spell of illness," as previously defined here. Consequently, rather than an annual deductible, the deductible is assessed at the beginning of each spell of illness. If a patient is hospitalized several times during a spell of illness, only one deductible is assessed. On the other hand, if a patient has multiple spells of illness in any given year, several deductibles may be charged. For example, about 15 percent of beneficiaries pay two or more deductibles in any given year. The size of the deductible increases each year at the same rate as Medicare payments to hospitals. In 1996 the deductible is $736. The historical trends in this and other beneficiary cost sharing are shown in table A.1.

Similarly, coinsurance is assessed on the basis of the number of covered days during a spell of illness. (The calculation of number of days may cumulate across multiple admissions to the hospital.) The first 60 days of hospital care require no coinsurance. Between days 61 and 90 of the spell of illness, the individual is assessed coinsurance of one-fourth the hospital deductible for each day (or $184 in 1996). After 90 days of hospitalization during a spell of illness, the Medicare beneficiary must draw upon a lifetime reserve of 60 additional days of coverage, while paying coinsurance equal to one-half the deductible ($368 in 1996) for each day. After exhausting that reserve, the Medicare beneficiary is liable for the full costs of any additional days in the hospital. About 0.5 percent of all Medicare enrollees exhaust their lifetime reserve days in any one year, usually because they have experienced several periods of hospitalization.

Coinsurance is also assessed on days 21 through 100 of a skilled nursing facility stay. The amount is set at one-eighth of the hospital deductible. At $92 in 1996, this amount is substantially larger than 20 percent, often totaling over half of what Medicare pays per day.

Consequently, many beneficiaries simply do not file for Medicare reimbursement for more than 20 days of SNF care.

In addition to the hospital deductible, there is another deductible equal to the cost of the first three pints of whole blood received by a beneficiary as part of covered inpatient services. This deductible is also calculated on a spell-of-illness basis. The patient can avoid this deductible by arranging for replacement of the blood by donors.

Finally, the hospice program requires several coinsurance payments. Beneficiaries must pay 5 percent coinsurance (up to $5) for each palliative drug and biological prescription furnished by the hospice when the beneficiary is *not* an inpatient. A 5 percent coinsurance payment is also required for each day of respite care, capped at the level of the hospital deductible.

Home health services do not require any cost sharing. A 20 percent coinsurance payment was required until 1973, when the bulk of home healthcare services were shifted to Part A from Part B.

Part B

Under Part B, the deductible is a set amount—now $100 per year—which does not rise automatically over time. It has been increased three times by legislation from an initial level of $50 per year. For physician and certain other services, the coinsurance is set at 20 percent of the amount that Medicare establishes as its "allowed" charge. Two major exceptions to the coinsurance requirement are clinical laboratory services, for which Medicare usually reimburses 100 percent of the fee schedule, and home health services. Most other services under Part B are subject to the coinsurance requirement. Since physician fees generally rise each year, the amount that Medicare beneficiaries pay in cost sharing consequently goes up even when the same level of services is used from year to year. On the other hand, coinsurance for outpatient services are much higher than 20 percent since they are based on charges and not on what Medicare pays.

The Part B premium is also tied to the costs of Part B services. Enrollees must pay approximately 25 percent of the costs of care for an elderly enrollee. That amount was first introduced as a temporary change in 1982 and has periodically been extended since then. In 1990–95, premium amounts were established using projected spending. In 1995, premiums covered about 31.5 percent of Part B costs. But in 1996 this share returned to 25% of costs, or $42.50 per month. This requirement will remain in force only through 1997 unless legislation extends it as has been done consistently since 1981.

Table A.1 MEDICARE DEDUCTIBLES, COINSURANCE, AND PREMIUMS, 1966–96

For Benefit Periods Beginning in Calendar Year	Inpatient Hospital			Skilled Nursing Facility, 21st-through 100th-Day Coinsurance ($)	Supplementary Medical Insurance Deductible ($)	Supplementary Medical Insurance Premium ($)
	First 60 Days' Deductible ($)	61st through 90th Day, Coinsurance per Day ($)	60 Lifetime Reserve Days ($)			
1966	40	10	—	—		
1967	40	10	—	5.00		
1968	40	10	20	5.00		
1969	44	11	22	5.50		
1970	52	13	26	6.50		
1971	60	15	30	7.50		
1972	68	17	34	8.50		
1973	72	18	36	9.00	50	3.00
1974	84	21	42	10.50	50	3.00
1975	92	23	46	11.50	50	4.00
1976	104	26	52	13.00	50	4.00
1977	124	31	62	15.50	50	5.30
1978	144	36	72	18.00	50	5.60
1979	160	40	80	20.00	50	5.80
					60	6.70
					60	6.70
					60	6.70
					60	7.20
					60	7.70
					60	8.20
					60	8.70

Year					
1980	180	45	90	22.50	60	9.60
1981	204	51	102	25.50	60	11.00
1982	260	65	130	32.50	75	12.20
1983	304	76	152	38.00	75	12.20
1984	356	89	178	44.50	75	14.60
1985	400	100	200	50.00	75	15.50
1986	492	123	246	61.50	75	15.50
1987	520	130	260	65.00	75	17.90
1988	540	135	270	67.50	75	24.80
1989[a]	560	NA	NA	25.50	75	31.90
1990	592	148	296	74.00	75	28.60
1991	628	157	314	78.50	100	29.90
1992	652	163	326	81.50	100	31.80
1993	676	169	338	84.50	100	36.60
1994	696	174	348	87.00	100	41.10
1995	716	179	358	89.50	100	46.10
1996	736	184	368	92.00	100	42.50

Source: Data from Health Care Financing Administration, Office of the Actuary, Office of Medicare Cost Estimates.
a. Includes MCCA legislation.

The original share that enrollees paid was higher, set at 50 percent in the enacting legislation. But over time, the premium grew much faster than Social Security payments, resulting in a Part B premium deduction from Social Security that was consuming an ever-increasing portion of monthly Social Security checks. The 1972 amendments to Medicare changed the premium so that thereafter it would grow no faster than the rate of the Social Security cost-of-living adjustment (COLA). Then the reverse problem arose. With high rates of healthcare spending in the 1970s, the share paid by beneficiaries gradually eroded to about 25 percent of Part B costs by 1981. The 1981 legislation essentially froze the premium share in place at 25 percent of the costs of an elderly enrollee as a federal budget reduction measure.

Normally the premium is automatically deducted from the beneficiary's Social Security check. Each January, both the Social Security COLA and the premium increase go into effect. An additional protection for beneficiaries with small monthly payment amounts is that for each enrollee, the Part B premium is not allowed to rise (in dollars) by an amount greater then the Social Security COLA. Consequently, whereas a few enrollees effectively have their COLA adjustment each year eliminated by the increase in Part B premiums, no one actually receives less in nominal dollars from one year to the next because of Medicare premium increases. And in practice, unless the Social Security COLA is very small and the Part B premium increase very large, only a few beneficiaries have their full COLA eliminated.[8]

GROWTH IN ENROLLEE LIABILITY

Since most of the cost sharing under Medicare is linked to expenditures, enrollees' liabilities have risen sharply over time. This is shown in figure A.1. Most of the liability comes from Part B, through coinsurance and the premium. Thus, although Part B is less expensive from the standpoint of federal dollars, it is the more costly program as far as beneficiaries are concerned. Ironically, hospital expenditures, which are less important for cost sharing, constitute the bulk of Medicare spending (figure A.2).

Paying Providers

Medicare providers must generally be certified as meeting certain standards. They then bill Medicare on a fee-for-service basis. Hospitals and other major providers do not, however, file each claim separately. Rather, they are paid periodically, with adjustments to reconcile the actual amounts they are owed. These periodic interim payments

Figure A.1 MEDICARE ENROLLEE COSTS

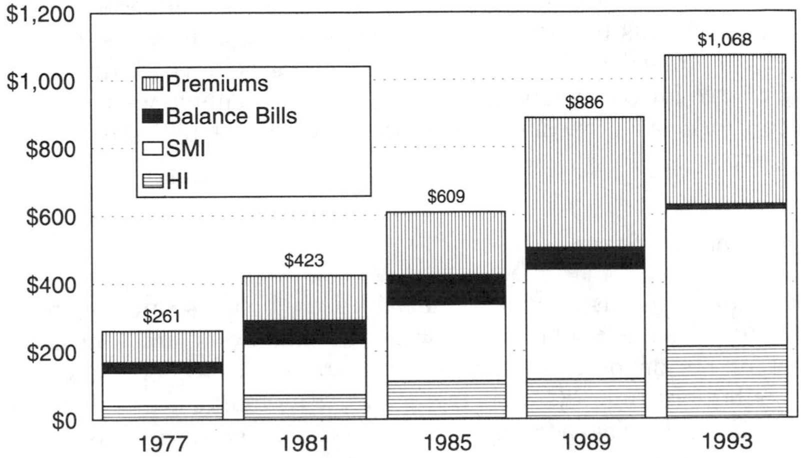

Source: Health Care Financing Review Statistical Supplement 1995.

(PIPs) were originally established to smooth the cash flow for hospitals. In the 1980s, they became a convenient, albeit bogus, device to achieve Medicare "savings." By delaying the payment from one fiscal year to the next, it can appear that Medicare had been cut.[9]

Physicians may ask patients to pay in full at the time of service, rather than seeking reimbursement from Medicare.[10] Physicians who directly bill Medicare are said to "accept assignment." If they accept assignment for all their Medicare patients, they are termed "participating providers" and are eligible for somewhat higher payments (allowed charges) for services. This distinction was made to encourage physicians to take assignment. If physicians decline to take assignment, they deal directly with the patient, who then must be reimbursed by Medicare. When such physicians bill their patients for more than the allowed charges, they are said to "balance bill" the patients, effectively asking patients to pay more than the formal coinsurance of 20 percent of allowed charges. Beginning in 1993, physicians were only allowed to charge no more than 115 percent of their approved charges, limiting any balance billing. The number of physicians seeking to balance bill their patients has declined rather dramatically over time. In 1980, 48.7 percent of all covered charges were balance billed; that percentage declined to 4 percent by 1994. The extent of balance billing varies by location of practice and specialty, however.

Over time, the calculations for paying hospitals, physicians, and other providers of Medicare services have become more and more complicated. Initially, payment policy for hospitals and other large providers was based simply on reported costs. In the case of physicians, payments reflected "reasonable charges," defined as the lower of either a physician's own usual or customary charge, or the prevailing charge for physicians in a particular area. This is where policies to control costs have concentrated; these issues are discussed in detail in chapter 3.

Financing the Program

Medicare Part A is financed almost entirely by a 1.45 percent tax on earnings, assessed of both employees and employers (and thus is a 2.9 percent tax on overall payroll). It is part of the Federal Insurance Contributions Act (FICA) tax that most individuals see as a deduction in their paychecks each pay period. It is assessed regardless of wage level on persons of all ages, but is paid mostly by persons under the age of 65 (since few persons over that age remain in the labor force). Medicare now differs from Social Security because there is no limit on earnings subject to Medicare's tax; Social Security's payroll tax is applied to only the first $62,700 of a worker's earnings in 1996. The payroll tax *rate* was last increased in 1986 as part of the 1983 Social Security amendments and is not currently scheduled to rise further.

Figure A.2 SHARE OF MEDICARE EXPENDITURES BY SERVICE

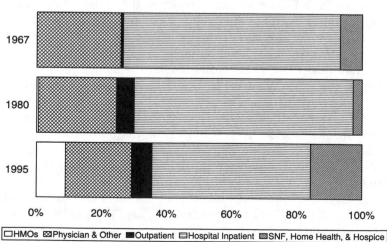

Source: CBO 1995; NCHS 1994.

In 1966, the initial tax rate was 0.7 percent (combined) against a base of $6,600 in earnings—for a maximum contribution of $46.20 per person that year. Today, there is effectively no limit since all earnings are subject to the tax. A worker with earnings of $200,000, for example, would have a total contribution (from both employee and employer contributions) of $5,800. A worker earning $30,000 per year would have a combined contribution of $870.

These revenues are combined with premiums (paid by those elderly not otherwise eligible), small general revenue transfers to cover beneficiaries such as railroad retirees, and interest from previous balances to form the Federal Hospital Insurance Trust Fund. Under the law, payments are made only so long as there is a positive balance in the trust fund. The HI trustees report for 1996 indicated a declining balance in the near term and total exhaustion of the trust fund by 2001 (see table A.2).

Part B's funding comes from the premium contributions of beneficiaries and general revenue contributions by the federal government. Although there is a trust fund for Part B as well as Part A, it is much less important since, by law, the U.S. Treasury must make up the difference between premium contributions and Part B spending. Thus, whereas general revenue contributions may be large, there is no crisis in funding requiring legislation, as is the case with Part A. But

Table A.2 ESTIMATED OPERATIONS OF FEDERAL HOSPITAL INSURANCE TRUST FUND, 1991–2002 ($ billions)

Calendar Year	Total Income (Billing, $)	Total Disbursements ($)	Net Increase in Fund ($)	Fund at End of Year ($)
1991	88.8	72.6	16.3	115.2
1992	93.8	85.0	8.8	124.0
1993	98.2	94.4	3.8	127.8
1994	109.6	104.5	5.0	132.8
1995	115.0	117.6	− 2.6	130.3
1996	120.3	129.5	− 9.2	121.0
1997	126.7	141.7	15.0	106.1
1998	130.2	154.5	− 24.3	81.8
1999	133.8	168.0	− 34.1	217.6
2000	137.5	182.2	− 44.7	3.0
2001	141.2	197.2	− 56.0	− 53.0
2002	145.5	213.1	− 67.6	− 120.7

Source: HI Trustees (1996).
Note: Data are based on Alternative II assumptions, which are usually considered intermediate assumptions regarding factors such as life expectancy and healthcare inflation.

Part B's growth has actually been higher than that for Part A in recent years, raising financing concerns for this part of Medicare as well.

Administering the Program

The Health Care Financing Administration (HCFA) is in charge of overseeing the Medicare program, and promulgates rules and regulations governing its operations. The administrative costs of the program are quite low overall—less than 2 percent of program outlays. Day-to-day processing of claims and oversight of providers is done at a much more disaggregated level, however. HCFA contracts with "fiscal intermediaries" to process Part A claims and contracts with "carriers" to process Part B claims. These groups, usually insurance companies, deal directly with hospitals and physicians, respectively, to determine the appropriate levels of payment and then pay those providers. These entities also check claims for accuracy and fraud, and provide summary records of healthcare use to HCFA.

Carriers and intermediaries have always had considerable latitude in interpreting HCFA instructions, often resulting in inconsistent enforcement of regulations. In turn, these actions affect whether beneficiaries have access to certain benefits. A good example is the skilled nursing benefit, which has been the subject of court cases to try to resolve some of the disparities. Even after such pressures, however, availability of skilled nursing facilities varies substantially across the country, likely reflecting differences in intermediaries' treatment as well as other factors.

In practice, HCFA's data have been rather incomplete in terms of what services have been provided and how much has been paid to providers, limiting the agency's ability to oversee the work of the carriers and intermediaries. Only in the last few years have carriers even been required to meet uniform reporting requirements. HCFA, however, has tried to improve data collection and reporting. For example, a new common working file project attempts to ensure that data are reported in a more consistent and reliable fashion. Regional centers now process information directly that used to be processed by the carriers and intermediaries and then passed on to HCFA.

HCFA also contracts with Peer Review Organizations (PROs) for further oversight of the use of services and quality control, particularly for hospital care. These organizations assess the appropriateness of care delivered, determine whether hospitalization was required, and, to a much lesser degree, assess the quality of that care. HCFA defines the mix of these activities in its scope of work for contractors, and these descriptions have changed over time. For example, in the third scope of work for the period 1988 to 1990, more attention was directed to assessing the quality of care. The tools for quality oversight are limited, however. For instance, when hospitals or physicians are found at fault, the main penalty available is exclusion from the Medicare program, leaving little room for intermediate remedies for less serious offenses. Further, many of the PROs' activities still center on cost-containment efforts. For example, retrospective reviews of a sample of inpatient hospital cases include generic quality screening, discharge review, admission review, review of invasive procedures, diagnosis-related group (DRG) validation, coverage review, and determination of the application of the waiver of liability provision (Lohr 1990).

Other activities to oversee the quality of care include certification of providers. For example, HCFA has its own process of certifying hospitals. In addition, it accepts certification of hospitals by the Joint Commission on Accreditation of Healthcare Organizations (JCAHO) in lieu of its own hospital certification process. This is referred to as "deemed status." Other providers have also sought deemed status if they meet accreditation standards established by their provider organizations.

Funding for research has always been part of HCFA's responsibilities as well. Recently, HCFA has broadened its interests to improve data, develop new measures for analysis, and spend additional funds on activities such as effectiveness research that may influence both the quality and cost of Medicare over time.

Notes

1. Unless otherwise noted, material for this appendix is drawn from several sources that detail the workings of the Medicare program. For more information, see Ways and Means (1992); Commerce Clearing House (1988); U.S. Social Security Administration (1991); HI Board of Trustees (1992); and SMI Board of Trustees (1992).

2. Coinsurance is a charge assessed against the user of a service that is defined as a percentage of the cost of that care. The term cost sharing normally refers to coinsurance and deductibles—the costs of care that beneficiaries are required to "share."

3. Technically, this is not coinsurance—although it is the term that Medicare uses—since it is not tied to the cost of SNF care, but, rather, to the cost of hospital services. This is described later in this appendix.

4. Home healthcare is also covered under Part B, but the only enrollees who receive home health through Part B now are those not also enrolled in Part A.

5. The dual, and essentially conflicting, requirements of intermittency and confinement to the home were criticized in the 1980s by elderly advocates as providing a "Catch 22" that precluded eligibility for many Medicare enrollees. Easing of the intermittency guidelines has lessened this problem and expanded use of this benefit dramatically in the 1990s.

6. The coinsurance requirements are extremely complicated in the case of hospital outpatient services. Although Medicare pays outpatient departments on the basis of costs, coinsurance is calculated on the basis of charges, which are generally higher. Consequently, most beneficiaries effectively pay more that 20 percent coinsurance for hospital outpatient facility services, and sometimes much more.

7. For example, the Part B premium is projected to increase $3.30 per month between 1996 and 1997. Assuming a COLA increase of 3 percent, only persons with benefits of less than $110 per month would have their COLAs fully eliminated. Only about 5.5 percent of retired workers receive payments of less than $250 per month.

8. In the budget agreements of 1981, 1982, and 1986, shifting of the timing of the (PIP) served as a major source of projected Medicare savings. In actuality, these efforts served to shift the timing of spending from one fiscal year to another and had no lasting effects on the federal budget deficit.

9. Even after the recent requirement that physicians must file claims for their patients, they can ask for payment directly from the beneficiary, rather than being paid by Medicare.

REFERENCES

American Association of Retired Persons/Public Policy Institute. 1995. *Coming Up Short: Increasing Out-of-Pocket Health Spending by Older Americans.* Washington, DC: Author, April.

American Hospital Association. 1995. *Hospital Statistics: 1995 Edition.* Chicago, IL: Author.

Bishop, Christine and Kathleen Carley Skwara. 1993. "Recent Growth of Medicare Home Health." *Health Affairs.* 10(Fall):95–110.

Board of Trustees, Federal Hospital Insurance Trust Fund. 1996. *1996 Annual Report of the Hospital Insurance Trust Fund.* Washington, DC: U.S. Government Printing Office.

_____. 1995. *1995 Annual Report of the Hospital Insurance Trust Fund.* Washington, DC: U.S. Government Printing Office.

_____. 1993. *1993 Annual Report of the Hospital Insurance Trust Fund.* Washington, DC: U.S. Government Printing Office.

_____. 1990. *1990 Annual Report of the Hospital Insurance Trust Fund.* Washington, DC: U.S. Government Printing Office.

Board of Trustees, Federal Supplementary Medical Insurance Fund. 1995. *1995 Annual Report of the Board of Trustees of the Federal Supplementary Medical Insurance Trust Fund.* Washington, DC: U.S. Government Printing Office.

Brown, Randall, Dolores Clement, Jerrold Hill, Sheldon Retchin, and Jeanette Bergeron. 1993. "Do Health Maintenance Organizations Work for Medicare?" *Health Care Financing Review.* 15(Fall):7–23.

Chesney, James D. 1990. "Utilization Trends before and after PPS." *Inquiry* 27(Winter):376–81.

Christensen, Sandra, and Rick Kasten. 1988. "Covering Catastrophic Expenses under Medicare." *Health Affairs* 7(Winter):79–93.

Chulis, George S., Franklin J. Eppig, Mary O. Hogan, Daniel R. Waldo, and Ross H. Arnett, III. 1993. "Health Insurance and the Elderly: Data from MCBS." *Health Care Financing Review.* 14(Spring):163–181.

Federal Register. 1995. "Medicare Program: Inpatient Hospital Deductible and Hospital and Extended Care Insurance Amounts for 1996." Vol. 60, October 16, 53625–53632.

Foster Higgins. 1995. *National Survey of Employer-Sponsored Health Plans/1994.* New York, NY: Author.

Gage, Barbara. 1995. "Medicare's Home Health Payments." Background material for Prospective Payment Assessment Commission, September 12. Photocopy.

Health Care Financing Administration. 1996a. "Average Annual Per Capita Costs (AAPCCs) under Medicare." Web site: http://www.hcfa.gov/.

————. Bureau of Data Management and Strategy. 1996b. Medicare Part A and B Enrollees by State.

————. 1996c. "List of Diagnosis Related Groups (DRGs) and Relative Weighting Factors." Web site: http://www.hcfa.gov/stats/stats.html/.

————. 1995. *Health Care Financing Review Statistical Supplement.* Baltimore, MD: Author, September.

Huskamp, Haiden and Joseph Newhouse. 1994. "Is Health Spending Slowing Down?" *Health Affairs.* 13(Winter):32–38.

Inspector General. 1995. *Beneficiary Perspectives of Medicare Risk HMOs.* OEI–06–91–00730. Washington, DC: U.S. Department of Health and Human Services.

Kenney, Genevieve and Marilyn Moon. 1996. "Medicare Home Health Growth and Options for Change." Report prepared for the Commonwealth Fund. Photocopy.

KPMG Peat Marwick. 1995. *Health Benefits in 1995.* Newark: Author.

————. 1994. *Health Benefits in 1994.* Newark: Author.

Lave, Judith. 1990. "The Impact of the Medicare Prospective Payment System and Recommendations for Change." *Yale Journal on Regulation* 7:499–528.

Loprest, Pamela. 1995. "Health Coverage of Early Retirees with Disabilities." Report to the Pension Welfare Benefits Administration, U.S. Department of Labor. Photocopy, June.

Lubitz, James, and Ronald Prihoda. 1984. "Use and Costs of Medicare Services in the Last Two Years of Life." *Health Care Financing Review* 5(Spring):117–31.

Lubitz, James D. and Gerald F. Riley. 1993. "Trends in Medicare Payments in the Last Year of Life." *New England Journal of Medicine.* 328:1092–6.

Miller, Mark, Stephen Zuckerman, and Michael Gates. 1993. "How Do Medicare Physician Fees Compare with Private Payers?" *Health Care Financing Review.* 14(Spring):25–39.

Mitchell, Janet, and Terri Menke. 1990. "How the Physician Fee Schedule Affects Medicare Patients' Out-of-Pocket Spending." *Inquiry* 27 (Summer):108–13.

Moon, Marilyn. 1996. "Understanding the Effects of Major Medicare Savings." Report prepared for the Commonwealth Fund. Photocopy, March.

————. 1994. "Lessons from Medicare." *The Gerontologist.* 34:606–611, October.

————. 1993. "Asset Limits and Medicaid." Urban Institute Working Paper. Washington, DC: The Urban Institute, April.

Moon, Marilyn and Janemarie Mulvey. 1996. "Incorporating Health and Asset Adjustments into Measures of Economic Well-Being." Urban Institute Discussion Paper #06402–01. Washington, DC: The Urban Institute, January.

_____. 1995. *Entitlements and the Elderly: Protecting Promises, Recognizing Realities.* Washington, DC: The Urban Institute Press.

Moon, Marilyn, Len Nichols, Korbin Liu, Genevieve Kenney, Margaret Sulvetta, Stephen Zuckerman, and Crystal Kuntz. 1995. "Searching for Savings in Medicare." Prepared for the Henry J. Kaiser Family Foundation, December. Photocopy.

Moon, Marilyn and Stephen Zuckerman. 1995. "Are Private Insurers Really Controlling Spending Better Than Medicare?" Henry J. Kaiser Family Foundation Discussion Paper, July. Photocopy.

National Center for Health Statistics. 1995. *Health United States 1994.* Hyattsville, MD: Public Health Service, May.

_____. 1991. *Health United States 1990.* Hyattsville, MD: Public Health Service.

Office of the President. 1996. *Budget of the United States Government, Fiscal Year 1997.* Washington, DC: U.S. Government Printing Office.

O'Sullivan, Jennifer. 1995. "Medicare: Financing the Part A Hospital Insurance Program." Congressional Research Service report to Congress. Washington, DC: Congressional Research Service, May. Photocopy.

Peterson, Peter G. 1993. *Facing Up: How to Rescue the Economy from Crushing Debt and Restore the American Dream.* New York, NY: Simon & Schuster.

Physician Payment Review Commission. 1996. *Annual Report to Congress.* Washington, DC: U.S. Government Printing Office.

_____. 1995. *Annual Report to Congress.* Washington, DC: U.S. Government Printing Office.

Prospective Payment Assessment Commission (ProPAC). 1996. *Medicare and the American Health Care System: Report and Recommendations to Congress.* Washington, DC: Author.

_____. 1995a. *Medicare and the American Health Care System: Report to Congress.* Washington, DC: Author, June.

_____. 1995b. *Medicare and the American Health Care System: Report and Recommendations to Congress.* Washington, DC: Author, March.

_____. 1993. *Medicare and the American Health Care System: Report to Congress.* Washington, DC: Author.

Rodgers, Jack and Karen E. Smith. "Is There Biased Selection in Medicare HMOs?" Report prepared for the Association of American Health Plans by Health Policy Economics Group, Price Waterhouse. Photocopy, March.

Rosenbach, Margo, Killard Adamache, and Rezaul Khandker. 1995. "Variations in Medicare Access and Satisfaction by Health Status: 1991–93" *Health Care Financing Review* 17(Winter):29–50.

Seib, Gerald. 1995. "How the GOP Seeks to Elude the Medicare Wreck." *The Wall Street Journal,* May 3:A16.

Social Security Administration. 1995. *Annual Statistical Supplement, 1995.* Washington, DC: Author, August.

U.S. Bureau of the Census. 1996. "Persons 15 Years Old and Over, by Median and Mean Income, and Sex." Web site http://www.census.gov/.

————. 1995a. "Income and Poverty: 1994 Poverty Summary." Web site http://www.census.gov/.

————. 1995b. *Asset Ownership of Households: 1993.* Current Population Reports, Series P-70, no. 47. Washington, DC: U.S. Government Printing Office.

————. 1995c. *Statistical Abstract of the United States: 1994 (114th edition).* Washington, DC: U.S. Government Printing Office.

————. 1995d. *Income, Poverty, and Valuation of Noncash Benefits: 1993.* Current Population Reports, Series P-60, no. 188. Washington, DC: U.S. Government Printing Office.

————. 1993. *Money Income of Households, Families and Persons in the United States: 1992.* Current Population Reports, Series P-60, No. 174. Washington, DC: U.S. Government Printing Office.

U.S. Congress, Committee on Ways and Means. 1994. *1994 Green Book: Overview of Entitlement Programs.* U.S. House of Representatives. Washington, DC: U.S. Government Printing Office.

U.S. Congressional Budget Office (CBO). 1996a. "Baseline: Medicare." Staff memorandum. Washington, DC: Author, April.

————. 1996b. "The Economic and Budget Outlook, Fiscal Years 1997–2006: A Preliminary Report." Washington, DC: Author, March.

————. 1994. "Reducing Entitlement Spending." Washington, DC: Author, September.

U.S. Department of Labor, Bureau of Labor Statistics. 1996. "Consumer Price Index-All Urban Consumers: All Items and Medical Care." Web site: http://stats.bls.gov/.

Wiener, Joshua M., Laurel Illston, and Raymond Hanley. 1994. *Sharing the Burden: Strategies for Public and Private Long-Term Care Insurance.* Washington, DC: The Brookings Institution.

Zuckerman, Stephen, Diana Verrilli, and Stephen Norton. 1996. Assessing the Viability of All-Payer Systems for Physician Services. Urban Institute Report #06375–01–06. Washington, DC: The Urban Institute, May.

ABOUT THE AUTHOR

Marilyn Moon is a Senior Fellow with the Health Policy Center of the Urban Institute. She has written extensively on health policy, policy for the elderly, and income distribution. She recently wrote *Entitlements and the Elderly: Protecting Promises, Recognizing Realities*, with Janemarie Mulvey (Urban Institute Press, 1995). Recent articles include "The Special Health Care Needs of the Elderly" and "Medical Savings Accounts: A Policy Analysis."

Marilyn Moon has also served as director of the Public Policy Institute of the American Association of Retired Persons. She has worked as a senior analyst in the Human Resources and Community Development Division of the Congressional Budget Office, and as associate professor of economics at the University of Wisconsin-Milwaukee. She was a consultant to the U.S. Bipartisan Commission for Comprehensive Health Care (the Pepper Commission) and is currently serving as one of the two public trustees of the Social Security and Medicare trust funds. She also writes an occasional column on health coverage for *The Washington Post*.

A

Access to benefits, 32, 38, 39, 41–42, 43, 105, 166
Acute care, 25n.2, 37, 89, 90, 98, 110, 130, 192, 193, 205–206, 213–215, 244
  costs of, 12
  coverage improvement, 235
  eligibility expansion, 200–204
  expansion of, 216
  expenses, 242–243
  prescription drugs and, 204–205
  QMB addition, 198–199
  stop-loss protection, 199–200
  supplemental coverage, 214
Adjusted average per capita cost (AAPCC), 83, 84, 156–157, 181, 194, 195, 245
Administration of program, 164, 165–166
Administrative costs, 12, 21, 66–68, 177–178, 192, 207, 224, 231, 254–255
Adverse selection issues, 203–204, 225, 235
Advisory Council on Social Security, 33
Age, 32
  eligibility, 188–192, 194, 195, 196n.11, 197–198, 216, 222, 233–234
  health insurance and, 201
  length of hospital stay and, 101

Agency for Health Care Policy and Research (AHCPR), 109
Allowed charges, 51
All-payer systems, 237n.2
Alternative care, 168
American Association of Retired Persons (AARP), 28, 31, 116, 119, 128, 149, 197
American Hospital Association, 17, 60–62
American Medical Association (AMA), 29, 30, 31, 32, 44n.7, 72, 153
Anderson, Clinton, 29
Assignment rates, 94–96
Association of American Physicians and Surgeons, 32
Average value of benefits, 194

B

Balance billing, 38, 94–97, 112n.7, 143n.8, 251
Balanced Budget Act of 1995, 1, 96–97, 112n.4, 149, 170n.6
Ball, Robert, 29
Beneficiaries
  benefits-contributions ratio, 33
  cost-containment, 159–164
  income/payment ratio, 159
  out-of-pocket expenses, 199
  PPS burden, 99–104
  provider to beneficiary ratio, 99
  vouchers, 176–179

Bentsen, Lloyd, 132–133
Billing issues, 166, 231
Birth rates, 10
Blacks, 130–131
Blue Cross/Blue Shield, 51, 116
Bowen Commission, 118–119
Bowen, Otis, 118–119
Brook, Robert, 109
Budget. see Federal budget
Bush, George, 2, 90, 134, 141, 148, 158, 182
Buy-ins, 44n.9, 127, 129, 203, 233
Byrnes, John, 31

C

Callahan, Daniel, 189
Capital costs, 86n.10
Capital spending, 152
Capitated plans, 71–72, 106, 156, 174, 175, 179–181
Carter, Jimmy, 52–53
Catastrophic coverage, 3–4, 12, 37, 43n.3, 82, 99, 111–112, 138, 164, 169–170, 170n.7, 176, 197, 200, 211, 216, 222, 235, 243
    financing of, 121–122
    legislative history, 118–122
    see also Medicare Catastrophic Coverage Act (MCCA)
Certification of providers, 255
Chesney, James, D., 104
Children, 143n.4
Chiropractors, 244
Choice of insurance, 233
Choice of plans, 174–176, 180, 218n.11
Choice of provider, 32
Christensen, Sandra, 37, 39
Chronic care, 37, 110
Chronic illnesses, 96
Claims, 113n.14, 250–252, 256n.10
    hospitals, 250–252
    processing of, 21, 32, 51–52, 354
Clinical laboratory services, 155, 247
Clinton, Bill, 148–149, 153, 174
    balanced budget, 1, 96–97, 112n.4
    budget reductions, 2

health care reform, 184, 220
COBRA protections, 201, 202, 203
Cohen, Wilbur, 29
Coinsurance, 31, 38, 92, 111, 112n.1, 116, 120, 126, 143n.6, 145–148, 154n.7, 181, 209–211, 243, 244, 255n.3
    hospital, 123, 182
    outpatient services, 256n.7
    Part A, 160, 194, 246–247
    Part B, 88n.27, 123–124, 127
    physicians, 247
    QMB program, 229–230
    SNF benefits, 123
COLA. see Cost-of-living-adjustment (COLA)
Colonial Penn, 31
Community hospitals, 56, 62, 65
Community-based services, 102, 236
Compulsory health insurance, 29
Congressional Budget Office, 46, 55, 87n.15, 121, 127, 132–133, 167, 187, 195
    insurance benefits, 129–130
    MCCA benefits, 131
Consumer price index (CPI), 14, 16, 47, 48, 112n.4
Consumer satisfaction, 109–111
Continuity of care, 179
Contributor-benefits ratio, 22, 23, 33
Conversion factor, 72, 76, 87n.21
Copayments, 95, 227, 244
    Part B, 137
Corry, Martin, 136
Cost containment, 35–36, 45, 110, 177
    impact on beneficiaries, 89–113
    providers, 223–224
    QMB program and, 229–230
    strategies for, 148–164
Cost sharing, 37, 89, 118, 199, 255n.3
    burdens of, 38–41
    catastrophic coverage and, 116–117
    changes in, 90–97
    Part A, 246–247
    Part B, 124–125, 247–250

restructuring of, 145–148
revision of, 226–228
SNF, 82
Cost-of-living adjustment (COLA),
44n.9, 93, 112n.8, 250, 256n.8
Counseling, 244
Cruikshank, Nelson, 29

D

Davis, Karen, 37
Death, health care and, 190–192
Deductibles, 38, 111, 112n.2, 116,
120, 140, 145–148, 170n.1, 195–
196n.1, 243, 244, 255n.3
  MCCA, 205
  Part A, 91–93, 127–128, 145–
148, 226–228, 246–247
  Part B, 44n.9, 49, 88n.26, 91–93,
98–99, 123–124, 127–128,
145–148, 159–161, 169, 182,
211–212, 226–228, 247–250
  physicians, 181
  prescription drugs, 126
  QMB program, 229–230
Delivery systems, 207–208
Demographics, 131
  age/length of hospital stay
relationship, 101
  changes in, 5, 9–10
  contributor-to-beneficiary ratio,
22, 23
  see also Age
Dependents, 217n.4, 242
Diagnosis-related group (DRG),
56–59, 60, 86n.6, 86n.8, 86n.9,
86n.14, 100, 151, 255
  adjustments to, 68–69
  mix changes, 63
Discrimination against Medicare
patients, 105
Disenrollment, 106
Disproportionate share, payments
to hospitals, 151–152
District of Columbia, 41
DRG. *see* Diagnosis-related group
(DRG)
Drugs. *see* Prescription drugs
Duggan v. *Bowen*, 79, 88n.28

Durable medical equipment, 18,
155, 245

E

Economic status of elderly, 5–13
Education campaigns, 158–159
Effectiveness studies, 108–109,
157–159
Eisenhower, Dwight, 28, 29
Eligibility, 31, 241–243
  age, 32, 101, 188–192, 194, 195,
196, 196n.11, 197–198, 201,
216, 222, 233–234
  disabled persons, 36
  expansion of, 200–204
  income, 192–193, 194, 196n.5,
196n.6, 199, 209
  means-testing, 192–193, 194
  public insurance, 212–213
  SS disability, 202
Emergency room services, 76, 77,
245
Employee fringe benefits, 229
Employer-provided coverage, 28–
29, 36, 112n.3, 117, 221
Employer-provided supplemental
coverage, 176
Employer-subsidized plans, 3, 7–8,
39, 183
Enrollees
  changes in, 35
  expenditures, 46–51
  growth of, 46–47
  HMOs, 82–84, 106–107, 155–157
  hospital admissions, 62
  income/out-of-pocket costs ratio,
129–130
  liability, 97, 111, 250, 251
  MAA, 27
  program complaints, 164–165
  use of services, 97–98
Enrollment cards, 164
Entitlements, 173–174, 187, 193
Episode-based payments, 155
Evaluation services, 73, 76, 77
Expenditures, 112n.1
  growth of, 76
  growth sources, 46–51

per beneficiary, 89–90
per capita, 116

F

Facility charges, 25n.9
Falk, I. S., 29
Federal budget, 90, 99, 148
  balanced, 196n.9
  deficit, 45–46, 143n.1, 144n.11
  Medicare growth and, 1–5
  Medicare share, 2–3, 20–21
  reductions, 53, 58
Federal Hospital Insurance Trust
  Fund, 2, 45, 253
Federal Insurance Contributions
  Act (FICA), 36, 234–235, 252–
  254
Federal Register, 72, 76
Federal workers, 36
Fee-for-service, 71–72, 175, 176,
  180, 224, 225, 235, 245, 250
Financing of Medicare, 252–254
Flemming, Arthur, 29
Forand, Aime, 29, 30
Fraud and abuse, 78, 149, 154, 254
Funding
  Part A, 20
  public share increase, 234–235

G

Geographic issues, 37–38, 41–42,
  58
  access to care, 105
  adjustments to, 74–75
  physician participation rate, 94
Geographic practice cost index
  (GPCI), 75
Geriatric care, 71
Goals of Medicare, 31–33
Government insurance program,
  212
Gramm-Rudman-Hollings bill, 115,
  143n.1
Great Society, 28, 29
Group health plans, 201, 202, 203

H

Hanley, Raymond, 12
Hawaii, 41
Health and Human Services
  Department, 55
Health Care Financing
  Administration (HCFA), 21, 33,
  37, 71–72, 74–76, 78, 84, 88n.28,
  105, 112n.6, 140, 152, 254–255
  balance billing estimates, 94
  capital costs, 86n.10
  conversion factor, 87n.21
  HMO participation expansion,
  224–226
  PRO contracts, 107–108
  quality of care issues, 106–107
Health care policy, 134–141
Health maintenance organizations
  (HMOs), 71, 82–84, 88n.29, 104,
  155–157, 174, 176, 177, 179–181,
  194
  Medicare expenditure, 252–253
  participation expansion, 224–
  226
  premiums, 245
  quality of care, 106–107, 226
High risk patients, 151–152
High-technology services, 73, 76,
  77
Home health care, 24–25n.1,
  25n.10, 77, 78–81, 85n.1, 102–
  103, 119–121, 123, 124, 137,
  143n.3, 166, 179, 206, 209–211,
  223–224, 244, 247, 256n.5
  age/use comparison, 97–98
  coinsurance, 145–148, 160–161,
  247
  costs of, 66–68
  Medicare expenditure, 252–253
  shift to Part B, 227, 229
  visits per user, 155
Homemaker services, 116
Hospice, 112n.5, 123, 124, 137, 155,
  164, 166–168, 244
  coinsurance, 247
  expansion of, 230–231
  Medicare expenditure, 252–253
Hospital care, 18, 24–25n.1, 46
Hospital Insurance. see Part A

Hospitals, 91–92, 221
admissions, 59–62, 87n.15, 103–104
ancillary departments, 86n.4
beneficiaries liability, 123
billing practices, 52
certification of, 255
claim filings, 250–252
coinsurance, 131, 160–161, 182, 226–228
cost containment, 150–153
cost sharing, 146–148
costs, 92, 200
deductibles, 160–162, 247
discharges, 32, 57–58, 111, 113n.9, 113n.12
disproportionate share of Medicare patients, 63–65, 69
empty beds, 60, 61
goods and services, 59, 63
length of stay, 25n.2, 31, 59–61, 92, 99–103, 103–104, 132, 181, 226, 243
lifetime limits on, 131
nursing staff, 62
payment system, 55–59, 223
personnel, 62–63
PPS and, 60–66, 84–85
preadmission screening, 146
private-pay patients, 207
readmission rates, 101–103
special care units, 86n.4
teaching, 56, 63–65, 69, 87n.17, 151–152
types, 56–57
see also Inpatient services; Outpatient services
Hsaio, William, 73–74

I

Illston, Laurel, 12
Immigrants, 242
Immunizations, 168, 245
Income
adjusted gross, 143n.5
benefits relationship, 39
cost sharing and, 39–41, 161–164
disabled persons, 202
diversity of, 230
eligibility and, 192–193, 194, 196n.5, 196n.6, 199
family, 8, 38–40
future prospects of, 9–10
geographic issues and, 41–42
growth in, 6
health care needs and, 43n.4
out-of-pocket expenses and, 12
per capita, 5–6, 189
percent spent on health care, 10
physicians, 14
premiums and, 121–122, 126–127
QMB program and, 200
use of services and, 38–40
Income tax, 185–187
Income-related cost sharing, 161–164, 192–193, 194, 196n.5
Income-related premiums, 170n.8, 171n.9, 183–186, 228–229
Indemnity insurance, 174
Independent practice association (IPA), 179
Indigent care, 151–152, 224, 225
Ineffective treatments, 221
Inflation, 14–16, 46, 49, 53, 63, 67, 153, 189
Inpatient services, 66–68, 87n.15, 103, 113n.13, 123, 124–125, 151, 244, 248–249
age/use comparison, 97–98
decrease in, 103–104
Medicare expenditure, 252–253
Institute of Medicine, 108
Insurance companies, 129, 196n.1, 221, 254
Intermittency of care, 79, 244
Internal Revenue Service (IRS), 122, 136, 143n.4
International Classification of Diseases, 86n.6

J

Johnson, Lyndon, 28, 29–30, 33
Joint Commission on Accreditation of Healthcare Organizations (JCAHO), 255

K

Kasten, Rick, 39
Kerr-Mills bill, 27, 30, 31
King, Cecil, 29
King-Anderson bill, 30

L

Labor force, 188, 242
Laboratory services, 78, 112n.5
Lave, Judith, 68
Legislative history, 28–31
Length of stay. see Hospitals,
    length of stay
Life expectancy, 37, 188
Life-prolonging technology, 167
Long, Russell, 31, 44n.6
Long-term care, 1, 4, 25n.2, 43–
    44n.5, 81, 102, 110, 118, 119–120,
    130, 137–138, 143n.2, 155, 175,
    177, 182, 212
    admissions, 204
    comprehensive coverage, 206–
        208
    costs of, 12
    expansion of, 236
    financing of, 216
    income-related benefits, 209
    Medicare expansion of, 209–211
    Medicare services, 211–212
    overview, 205–206
    public insurance, 212–213
    two-track option, 213–215
Lubitz, James, 190

M

MAA. see Medical Assistance to
    the Aged (MAA)
MAAC. see Maximum allowable
    actual charge (MAAC)
Malpractice, 75
Mammography, 77, 125, 126, 137,
    168
Managed care, 82–84, 155–157,
    174, 175, 176, 180, 180–181, 221
    expansion of, 224–226
Management services, 73, 76, 77
Market basket, 150

Maximum allowable actual charge
    (MAAC), 94
Means-tested health care, 30,
    43n.3, 44n.6
Means-testing, 120, 140–141, 142,
    170n.8, 187, 192–193, 194,
    196n.5, 196n.6
Medicaid, 12, 31–32, 37, 43–44n.5,
    87n.17, 112n.3, 120–121, 126, 132,
    134, 159, 162, 196n.4, 196n.7,
    207, 208, 210, 211, 217n.1, 217n.3,
    230
    benefits, 198
    buy-ins, 127, 129
    cost sharing and, 39
    criticism of, 217n.8
    drug benefits, 204
    eligibility requirements, 39
    long-term care and, 205–206
    payment methods, 59
    poverty and, 25n.3
    spousal protection, 137
    supplemental acute care
        benefits, 198–199
Medical Assistance to the Aged
    (MAA), 27, 30, 31, 43n.2, 43n.5
Medical education, 224, 225
Medical price index, 16, 85n.1
Medical savings accounts (MSA),
    176, 195–196n.1
Medical social services, 244
Medical supplies, 244
Medicare Catastrophic Coverage
    Act (MCCA), 3–4, 12, 43n.3, 82,
    111–112, 118, 164, 169–170,
    170n.7, 197, 200, 216, 243
    benefits, 124–125
    coinsurance, 205
    deductibles, 205
    health policy and, 142–143
    impact of, 127–128
    income-related costs, 161–164
    Medicaid to Medicare shift, 198
    Medicare's future and, 137–141
    passage of, 122–133
    prescription drugs, 205
    preventive services, 168
    repeal of, 133–134
    SNF changes, 210, 211
    supplemental premium, 135–137

Medicare Economic Index (MEI), 49–51, 85n.3
Medicare Fee Schedule, 72–77, 104, 105, 153, 154
Medigap, 10–12, 41, 92, 116, 117, 127–130, 138–139, 144n.12, 182, 183, 204, 235
MEI. *see* Medicare Economic Index (MEI)
Men
    MCCA and, 130
    Medicare use, 37
Menke, Terri, 112n.7
Mental health services, 175, 244
Mills, Wilbur, 29–30, 31
Minority groups, 37–38, 139
Mitchell, Janet, 96, 112n.7
Mortality rates, 101–103
Myers, Robert, 45, 52

N

National Center for Health Services Research, 109
National Committee to Preserve Social Security, 143n.10
National Council of Senior Citizens, 29, 31
National health insurance, 28, 35
New York Times, 32, 44n.7
Nixon, Richard, 33, 45
Nonemployer insurance coverage, 201
Nongroup coverage, 201
Nonsurgical services, 75, 154
Nonteaching hospitals, 65
Nursing homes, 12, 77, 82, 102, 116, 206, 210, 217n.7, 236

O

Occupational therapy, 244
Office of Management and Budget (OMB), 134, 144n.11
Old Age Assistance, 43n.1
Omnibus Budget Reconciliation Act of 1981, 53
Omnibus Budget Reconciliation Act of 1986, 92

Omnibus Budget Reconciliation Act of 1989, 72
Omnibus Budget Reconciliation Act of 1990, 168, 243
Out-of-pocket spending, 7–8
Out-of-pocket expenses, 11, 12, 13, 37, 39, 43, 89, 93, 96, 116–117, 118, 121, 127, 129–130, 138, 193, 199–200
    age variations, 98
    hospital use ratio, 117
    prescription drugs, 205
Outpatient services, 60, 67–68, 77, 78, 85n.1, 103, 113n.13, 152–153, 179, 223–224, 245
    coinsurance, 256n.7
    Medicare expenditure, 252–253
Oversight protection, 166, 226, 254–255

P

Pain alleviation, 244
Part A, 24–25n.1, 88n.27, 102, 170n.2, 242
    beneficiaries liability, 123, 200
    benefits, 124–125, 226–228, 229, 243–244
    buy-in, 44n.9
    claims, 254
    coinsurance, 147, 160, 194, 246–247
    cost sharing, 118, 246–247
    deductibles, 38, 91–93, 127–128, 145–148, 226–228, 246–247
    enrollee costs, 251
    enrollee growth/service use relationship, 47
    funding, 20, 21–22, 25n.12, 252–253
    funds depletion, 173
    growth of, 52–54, 66–68
    heaviest users, 97–98
    home health services, 79, 80
    income-related premium, 163
    inflation impact, 47–49
    premiums, 147, 217n.9, 228–229
    trust fund, 66, 67, 228–229
    see also Services

Part B, 24–25n.1, 31, 32, 71, 88n.27,
    242, 256n.5
  age/use comparison, 98
  benefits, 124–125, 244–245
  claims, 254
  coinsurance, 127
  copayments, 95, 137
  cost sharing, 118, 247–250
  cost to beneficiaries, 135–136
  deductibles, 38, 44n.9, 49, 91–
    93, 98–99, 127–128, 145–148,
    159–161, 169, 182, 211–212,
    226–228, 247–250
  drug benefits, 140
  enrollee costs, 251
  funding, 253–254
  home health addition, 227, 229
  income-related cost, 162–163
  out-of-pocket expenses, 119–121,
    126
  premiums, 37, 112n.8, 118, 147,
    159–161, 170n.2, 183, 184, 194,
    196n.2, 199, 211–212, 237n.4,
    247
  subsidies, 122
Part C, 143n.3, 211, 235
Patient records, 179
Payroll taxes, 20, 21, 25n.12, 32,
    36, 173, 177, 234–235, 252–254
Peer Review Organizations (PROs),
    60, 107–108, 254–255
Pensions, 9, 201
Pepper, Claude, 120, 137, 143n.3
Pepper Commission, 210, 236,
    238n.7
Periodic interim payments, 250–
    252, 256n.9
Peterson, Peter, 170n.8, 196n.6
Pharmaceutical Manufacturers
    Association, 129, 131, 143n.10
Physical therapy, 79, 244, 245
Physician Payment Review
    Commission (PPRC), 71, 87n.24
Physician services, 24–25n.1,
    25n.2, 38, 93, 244
  age/use comparison, 97–98
  prices of, 44n.7
  volume of, 221
Physicians
  assignment of payment, 251

billing practices, 51, 75, 94–97,
    112n.7, 143n.8, 251
  business volume, 105
  charges, 25n.9, 85n.3, 244–245
  coinsurance, 247
  cost sharing, 98
  cost-containment, 153–154
  cross-specialty services, 74
  deductibles, 181
  fee freeze, 69–71, 87n.19, 93–94
  growth in services, 153
  home health services, 244
  malpractice, 75
  Medicare expenditures, 252–253
  office visits, 77, 96
  payment limit, 123
  payment reform, 69–77, 85, 94–
    97, 105
  payment system, 17, 49–51, 153,
    223, 251, 256n.10
  payment/quality of care
    relationship, 105
  political presence, 153
  services, 67–68
  specialties, 16, 17, 74, 94, 153,
    180
  supply of, 14
  volume performance standards,
    75
Point-of-service, 164, 166
Politics and health care, 28–30,
    31–32, 55, 69–72, 78, 119–121,
    126, 133–134, 135, 153, 192–193,
    194, 208, 209, 220, 222
Pope, Gregory, 75
Population, aging of, 189–190, 220
Postacute care, 67
Postoperative infections, 100
Poverty, 37, 39
  elderly, 6–8
  guidelines, 199
  health care coverage, 43n.4
  MCCA and, 130
  rates of, 25n.3, 27
PPRC. see Physician Payment
    Review Commission (PPRC)
PPS. see Prospective Payment
    System (PPS)
Preferred provider organizations
    (PPOs), 176, 177, 179

Premiums, 38, 111, 118–119, 121, 243
  actuarially fair, 241–242
  HMOs, 225, 245
  income-related, 121, 122, 126–127, 141, 183–186
  increase in, 183–185, 199
  Part A, 217n.9
  Part B, 37, 112n.8, 147, 159–161, 170n.2, 194, 196n.2, 199, 211–212, 237n.4, 247
  Part C, 235
  progressive, 237n.4
  QMB programs 229
  sliding scale, 237n.4
  supplemental, 121–122, 126–127, 132–133, 135–137, 217n.3, 243
Prescription drugs, 110–111, 116, 117, 120, 121, 125–126, 132–133, 137, 140, 177, 193, 197, 204–205, 216, 217n.1, 220, 235, 245, 247
  cost of, 17
  deductibles, 126
Preventive services, 165, 168–169, 177, 179
Prihoda, Ronald, 190
Primary care services, 76, 77
Privacy issues, 166
Private insurance, 18, 27, 28, 36, 51, 65, 84, 91, 130, 139, 144n.12, 154, 176–179, 179, 182, 195, 201, 206, 208, 212, 218n.10, 221, 231, 233, 242–243
Private supplemental insurance, 10–12, 116, 117, 121, 142, 165, 204
Private supplemental insurance, 176
Private-pay patients, 207
Privatized system, 1, 4–5
Productivity, 14
Professional Standards Review Organizations (PSROs), 52, 113n.15
ProPAC. see Prospective Payment Assessment Commission (ProPAC)
Proportional tax, 219
PROs. see Peer Review Organizations (PROs)

Prospective Payment Assessment Commission (ProPAC), 55, 86n.13
Prospective payment input price index, 59, 63
Prospective Payment System (PPS), 53, 55, 86n.7, 86n.10, 86n.12, 86n.13, 87n.15, 89, 146, 150–151, 152–153, 154
  adjustments to, 58
  admissions and, 59–60, 61
  condition of patients and, 104
  costs growth, 84–85
  deductibles, 92
  home health services, 155
  hospital admissions and, 103–104
  hospital discharges and, 113n.10
  hospital personnel and, 62–63
  impact of, 60–68, 101–103, 112n.2
  length of stay and, 59–61
  Medicare Fee Schedule and, 72
  modifications to, 68–69
  operating margins, 63–66
  overview, 55–59
  quality of care and, 104
Provider payments, 154–155, 223
Providers
  certification of, 255
  payments to, 250–252
  PSROs. see Professional Standards Review Organizations (PSROs)
  Psychiatric services, 243
  Psychoses, 86n.9
  Public insurance, 212–213

Q

Qualified Medicare Beneficiary (QMB), 12, 37, 39, 99, 138, 161–164, 183–186, 196n.4, 196n.5, 196n.7, 216, 243
  expansion of, 229–230
  shift to Medicare, 198–199
  stop-loss protection, 200
Quality of care, 62, 75, 100, 104–111, 150, 158, 207, 254–255

HMOs, 226
Quality of life, 18, 236

R

Racial issues, 38
RAND Corporation, 38, 101, 108, 158
Reagan, Ronald, 36, 55, 90, 91, 135, 148
budget reductions, 2
catastrophic coverage, 118, 123
fee schedules, 71
Medicare benefits, 115
Medicare cuts, 45–46
Medicare expansion, 118–119
tax policy, 136, 137
Regulation, 178
Rehabilitation services, 209–211, 244
Reinsurance, 183
Relative value scale, 153–154
Relative value units (RVUs), 73–74
Resource-based relative value scale (RBRVS), 71–72, 73–75, 85
Respiratory infections, 86n.9
Respite care, 125, 137, 244
Retirees, 200, 222
benefits, 27, 117, 188
coverage, 25n.6
earnings, 33
health insurance, 201–202
supplemental insurance, 39–41
Retirement age, 10
Riley, Gerald F., 190
Risk adjustment system, 225–226
Risk sharing, 174–176, 177, 178, 179, 181, 196n.1, 207, 215, 236
Rostenkowski, Dan, 133
Rural areas, 41, 71, 96
Rural health clinic services, 245
Rural hospitals, 63–65

S

Sanctions, 107
Secondary payers, 36, 242
Senior Coalition Against the Tax, 135

Services
age determination for, 189
changes in, 211–212
exclusion of, 110
growth of, 19, 47–49
overuse of, 109
preventive, 165, 168–169, 177, 179
underuse of, 158
use of, 16–20, 39, 46, 47, 77, 145–148, 164, 224
see also Home health services; Procedures and tests
Skilled nursing care, 24–25n.1, 25n.10, 31, 66–68, 85n.1, 102, 146–147, 155, 166, 209–211, 226–227, 244, 254
age/use comparison, 97–98
Skilled nursing facility (SNF), 47, 66–68, 78, 81–82, 88n.27, 91–92, 97–98, 102–103, 119–121, 123, 124, 132, 137–138, 140, 143n.9, 181, 209–211, 223–224, 243–244, 246–247
coinsurance, 145–148, 160–161, 164, 226–228, 247–248
cost-sharing, 146–148
Medicare expenditure, 252–253
Sliding scale premium payment, 199
Social insurance, 29, 30, 206
Social Security, 25n.12, 25n.13, 29, 149, 163, 171n.9, 187, 196n.7, 200, 217n.3, 236, 237n.4, 242
administrative costs, 207
benefits growth, 9
cost-of-living adjustment, 44n.9, 93, 112n.8, 250, 256n.8
disability benefits, 13, 25n.7, 213
disabled persons, 33–35, 36, 202
eligibility for, 241
federal workers and, 36
growth in benefits, 93
Medicare eligibility and, 33–34
Medicare premiums and, 250
solvency of, 55
taxation of benefits, 228–229, 234

Social Security Administration, 242
Social Security amendments, 93, 113n.15, 188
Socialized medicine, 32, 51
Specified Low Income Medicare Beneficiary Program (SLMB), 12, 39, 190–199, 229, 243
Speech therapy, 79, 245
Spells of illness, 143n.6, 148, 226, 243, 246–247
Spend down, 205–206, 217n.6
Spousal impoverishment provisions, 120, 137
Standard of living, 12
Stason, William, 73–74
Step-down care, 102, 104
Stop-loss protection, 126, 199–200, 235
Subsidies, 203–204, 212, 218n.10, 222, 224, 225, 242
   Part B, 122
   teaching hospitals, 69
Sullivan, Louis, 165
Supplemental coverage, 10–12, 13, 39–41, 113n.14, 222
Supplemental Medical Insurance (SMI). *see* Part B
Supplemental premiums, 121–122, 126–127, 132–133, 135–137
Supplemental Security Income, 217n.3, 243
Surgical services, 17–18, 73, 75, 76, 77, 154, 157–159
   risks of, 18
   unnecessary, 108–109

T

Tax Equity and Fiscal Responsibility Act (TEFRA), 36, 53–55, 86n.5, 69
Taxation, 163, 237n.1
   benefits, 185–187, 222
   FICA, 35, 234–235, 252–254
   income-related premiums, 228
   increase in, 236
   proportional tax, 219

Social Security benefits, 228–229, 234
surtax, 136
see also Payroll taxes
Teaching hospitals, 56, 63–65, 69, 87n.17, 151–152
Technologies, 104, 189–190 ·
TEFRA. *see* Tax Equity and Fiscal Responsibility Act (TEFRA)
Terminally ill, 112n.5, 166–168, 192
Third party payers, 16
Treasury Department, 132
Truman, Harry, 28
Trust fund, 20, 25n.13, 32–33, 45
   assets, 23
   future of, 21–22
223 limit, 52, 53

U

Underserved areas, 41–42, 43, 105
Unemployment, 202
Uninsured, 143n.2, 234
Unions, 31, 128
Universal coverage, 30, 43, 192–193, 205, 207–208, 222
Urban areas, 41–42
Urban hospitals, 63–65

V

Vision care, 116
Volume performance standard (VPS), 75, 154
Vouchers, 174, 176–179, 195, 194, 233

W

Warren, Earl, 29
Women
   insurance coverage, 201
   MCCA and, 130
   Medicare use, 37
   pregnant, 143n.4
Workplace issues, 13

1776